Bronchoalveolar Lavage in Basic Research and Clinical Medicine

This book provides a practical approach to bronchoalveolar lavage (BAL) and its analyses, which are used worldwide in both research and clinical settings. It includes useful guidelines with a theoretic background and provides details on microscopic and flow cytometric measurements for all known differential diagnostics made with BAL analyses, from chronic diseases like COPD and ILD via infectious diseases to inherited illnesses like cystic fibrosis. It includes BAL in both adult and pediatric medicine. The text is supported throughout by illustrations and clinical cases, serving as an invaluable resource for respiratory medicine and infectious disease clinicians and trainees.

Key features

- Uses BAL in the infectious diseases field and the search for respiratory viruses using the reverse transcription polymerase chain reaction (RT-PCR) technique.
- Presents contributions from worldwide experts.
- Clarifies the BAL technique and its diagnostic utility to respiratory physicians, cytologists, and pathologists involved in the diagnosis of pulmonary disease.
- Provides an updated perspective on the future applications of BAL technology to research and clinical medicine.

Bronchoalveolar Lavage in Basic Research and Clinical Medicine

Edited by

Oliver Schildgen
Prof. Dr rer.nat. Oliver Schildgen
Head of Molecular Pathology Division
Institute of Pathology, University Hospital of Witten/Herdecke Private University,
Hospital of the City of Cologne, Germany (Kliniken der Stadt Köln)

Verena Schildgen
Priv.-Doz. Dr rer.nat. Verena Schildgen
Lecturer for Molecular Pathology
Institute of Pathology, University Hospital of Witten/Herdecke Private University,
Hospital of the City of Cologne, Germany (Kliniken der Stadt Köln)

Michael Brockmann
Prof. Dr med. Michael Brockmann
Director and Chief Pathologist
Institute of Pathology, University Hospital of Witten/Herdecke Private University,
Hospital of the City of Cologne, Germany (Kliniken der Stadt Köln)

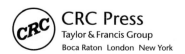

CRC Press
Taylor & Francis Group
Boca Raton London New York

CRC Press is an imprint of the
Taylor & Francis Group, an **informa** business

Cover image: Shutterstock ID 1596844453

First edition published 2024
by CRC Press
2385 NW Executive Center Drive, Suite 320, Boca Raton FL 33431

and by CRC Press
4 Park Square, Milton Park, Abingdon, Oxon, OX14 4RN

CRC Press is an imprint of Taylor & Francis Group, LLC
© 2024 Taylor & Francis Group, LLC

ISBN: 9780367705435 (hbk)
ISBN: 9780367705428 (pbk)
ISBN: 9781003146834 (ebk)

DOI:10.1201/ 9781003146834

Typeset in Minion
by Deanta Global Publishing Services, Chennai, India

Contents

Preface

Laughing is for the soul, what oxygen is for the lungs.

Louis de Funès

Salad bars are like a restaurant's lungs. They soak up the impurities and bacteria in the environment, leaving you with much cleaner air to enjoy.

Douglas Coupland, Brainyquote.com, "Bacteria Quotes," 19 July 2023

Editors

Oliver Schildgen

Prof. Dr rer. nat. Oliver Schildgen is the head of the Molecular Pathology Division within the Institute of Pathology at the University Hospital of Witten/Herdecke Private University at the Hospital of the City of Cologne, Germany. He holds a diploma in biology and earned his PhD at the University Hospital in Essen under the supervision of Michael Roggendorf before he joined the Institute for Microbiology and Immunology at the University of Bonn (meanwhile Institute of Virology) and the herpes virus research group of Bertfried Matz. After his habilitation in virology in 2006, he is now Professor of Virology and a certified clinical virologist (GfV). Following the scientific career started in clinical and applied virology Dr Schildgen switched to the field of molecular pathology and together with his team established the molecular unit within the Institute of Pathology. His research interests are newly discovered respiratory viruses, especially human bocavirus, viral DNA replication, and the interaction of respiratory viruses with solid tumors. Dr Schildgen has received several national and international scientific awards and is active as editor-in-chief for *Reviews and Research in Medical Microbiology*, section editor for microbiology of *Medicine*, and as scientific editor for several other journals.

Michael Brockmann

Prof. Dr med. Michael Brockmann has been the director and chief pathologist of the Institute of Pathology at the University Hospital of Witten/ Herdecke Private University at the Hospital of the City of Cologne, Germany, since 1996. He is Professor of Pathology at Witten/Herdecke Private University. His career as a pathologist started in Minden under the supervision of Prof. Dr W Busanny-Caspari and Dr E Jehn after which he joined the Institute of Pathology at the Bergmannsheil Bochum Hospital (i.e., University Hospital Bochum) and the group of Prof. Dr K-M Müller. At that time, he was mainly involved in establishing the national mesothelioma register. Dr Brockmann specializes in the pathology of lower respiratory tract diseases. He established the diagnostic BALF analyses in Cologne and serves as chief pathologist for several cancer centers in the Cologne area.

Verena Schildgen

Dr rer. nat. Verena Schildgen has a diploma in biology and is private lecturer (Privat-Dozentin) for Molecular Pathology. After finishing her diploma in Cologne and a research term in the Department of Immunogenetics at the University of Bonn, she presented her PhD thesis on myelodysplatics syndromes at the Heinrich Heine University in Düsseldorf, before joining the Institute of Pathology at the University Hospital of Witten/Herdecke Private University at the Hospital of the City of Cologne, Germany, where she is involved in molecular diagnostics and leads several research projects on acute and chronic respiratory disease complexes. Her research interests are immunology, cell biology, and molecular pathology of solid tumors and airway diseases.

For her research work on respiratory diseases, she has received three international scientific awards, i.e., the Rudolf Schülke Award, the Science Award of the Deutschsprachige Mykologische Gesellschaft (2014 in Salzburg, Austria), and the Wolfgang-Stille-Award of the Paul-Ehrlich-Society (PEG) for Chemotherapy (together with Oliver Schildgen).

List of Contributors

Jane Baer
Advance Diagnostics Laboratory
National Jewish Health
Denver, Colorado, USA

Elena Bargagli
Department of Medicine, Surgery, and
Neuroscience
University of Siena
Siena, Italy

Laura Bergantini
Department of Medicine, Surgery, and
Neuroscience
University of Siena
Siena, Italy

Parminder Singh Bhomra
University Hospitals Birmingham NHS
Foundation Trust
Institute of Applied Health Research
University of Birmingham, UK

Francesco Bonella
Department of Pneumology
Ruhrlandklinik University Hospital
University of Duisburg-Essen
Essen, Germany

Bryan Borg
Division of Pulmonary Sciences and Critical Care
Medicine
University of Colorado Anschutz Medical
Campus
Aurora, Colorado, USA
and
Department of Medicine
Rocky Mountain Regional Veterans Affairs
Medical Center
Aurora, Colorado, USA

Paolo Cameli
Department of Medicine, Surgery, and
Neuroscience
University of Siena
Siena, Italy

Stefano Cattelan
Department of Medicine, Surgery, and
Neuroscience
University of Siena
Siena, Italy

Edward D Chan
Division of Pulmonary Sciences and Critical Care
Medicine
University of Colorado Anschutz Medical
Campus
Aurora, Colorado, USA
and
Department of Medicine
Rocky Mountain Regional Veterans Affairs
Medical Center
Aurora, Colorado, USA
and
Department of Academic Affairs
National Jewish Health
Denver, Colorado, USA

Pierre Chauvin
Department of Respiratory Medicine
CHU Rennes
Rennes, France
and
IRSET UMR1085
University of Rennes
Rennes, France

Ulrich Costabel
Department of Pneumology
Ruhrlandklinik University Hospital
University of Duisburg-Essen
Essen, Germany

Miriana d'Alessandro
Department of Medicine, Surgery, and
Neuroscience
University of Siena
Siena, Italy

Emily Decurtis
Molecular Diagnostics
University of Colorado Anschutz Medical
Campus
Aurora, Colorado, USA

Bertrand De Latour
Department of Cardiothoracic Surgery
CHU Rennes
Rennes, France

Etienne Delaval
Department of Cardiothoracic Surgery
CHU Rennes
Rennes, France

Joanna Domagała-Kulawik
Maria Curie-Sklodowska Medical Academy
Institute of Clinical Sciences
Warsaw, Poland

Erwan Flecher
Department of Cardiothoracic Surgery
CHU Rennes
Rennes, France

Amy Frey
Department of Pathology
University of Colorado Anschutz Medical
Campus
Aurora, Colorado, USA

Marco Guerrieri
Department of Medicine, Surgery, and
Neuroscience
University of Siena
Siena, Italy

Josune Guzman
General and Experimental Pathology
Ruhr University Bochum
Bochum, Germany

Lutz-Bernhard Jehn
Department of Pneumology
Ruhrlandklinik University Hospital
University of Duisburg-Essen
Essen, Germany

Stéphane Jouneau
Department of Respiratory Medicine
CHU Rennes
Rennes, France
and
IRSET UMR1085
University of Rennes
Rennes, France

Samantha King
Division of Pulmonary Sciences and Critical Care
Medicine
University of Colorado Anschutz Medical
Campus
Aurora, Colorado, USA

Mallorie Kerjouan
Department of Respiratory Medicine
CHU Rennes
Rennes, France

Michael Kreuter
Center for Interstitial and Rare Lung Diseases
University of Heidelberg
Heidelberg, Germany

Terri Lebo
Immunology Laboratory
University of Colorado Anschutz Medical
Campus
Aurora, Colorado, USA

Mathieu Lederlin
Department of Radiology
CHU Rennes
Rennes, France
and
LTSI, INSERM U1099
University of Rennes
Rennes, France

Adel Maamar
Department of Infectious Diseases and Medical
Resuscitation
CHU Rennes
Rennes, France

Cédric Ménard
Department of Immunology, Cell Therapy, and
Hematopoiesis
Hôpital Pontchaillou
Rennes, France

Danielle Munce
Division of Pediatric Pulmonology
Rady Children's Hospital, University of California
San Diego
San Diego, California, USA

Benoit Painvin
Department of Infectious Diseases and Medical
Resuscitation
CHU Rennes
Rennes, France

Aparna Rao
Division of Pediatric Pulmonology
Rady Children's Hospital, University of California
San Diego
San Diego, California, USA

Mona Rizeq
Department of Pathology
University of Colorado Anschutz Medical
Campus
Aurora, Colorado, USA

Annegret Schlimbach
Institute of Pathology
Witten/Herdecke Private University
Cologne, Germany

Nicolaus Schwerk
German Center for Lung Research
Hanover Medical School
Hanover, Germany

Daniella Spittle
University Hospitals Birmingham NHS
Foundation Trust,
Institute of Applied Health Research,
University of Birmingham, UK

Tobias Stahlhut
Institute of Pathology
Witten/Herdecke Private University
Cologne, Germany

Florian Stehling
Department of Pediatrics
Universitätsklinikum Essen
Essen, Germany

Kelan Tantisira
Division of Pediatric Pulmonology
Rady Children's Hospital, University of California
San Diego
San Diego, California, USA

Jena Tisdale
Microbiology Laboratory
University of Colorado Anschutz Medical
Campus
Aurora, Colorado, USA

Alice M Turner
University Hospitals Birmingham NHS
Foundation Trust,
Institute of Applied Health Research,
University of Birmingham, UK

Vanessa Vedder
Institute of Pathology
Witten/Herdecke Private University
Cologne, Germany

Dehua Wang
Division of Pediatric Pathology
Rady Children's Hospital, University of California
San Diego
San Diego, California, USA

YongBao Wang
Molecular Diagnostics
University of Colorado Anschutz Medical
Campus
Aurora, Colorado, USA

Richard Wong
Division of Pediatric Pulmonology
Rady Children's Hospital, University of California
San Diego, California, USA

PART 1

Performing and analyzing BAL
(focus on technical aspects)

Bronchoalveolar lavage: A short introduction, historical aspects, frequent cytological observations, and basic laboratory protocols

OLIVER SCHILDGEN, TOBIAS STAHLHUT, ANNEGRET SCHLIMBACH, MICHAEL BROCKMANN, AND VERENA SCHILDGEN

The bronchoalveolar lavage (BAL) and the subsequent diagnostics of the recovered BAL fluid (BALF) have been established as an important clinical tool that is accepted for complex diagnostics of the lower airways. Its diagnostic usage enables the differential diagnosis of the most common interstitial lung diseases (ILDs). The BAL provides fluid specimens from the alveolar space and therefore should be differentiated from the bronchial lavage, which flushes only the bronchial tubes and is also used for therapeutic reasons like removing mucus.

However, this distinction is not always consistent. Especially at the beginning when the BAL was implemented as a lower respiratory tract sampling method (1) and in the 1990s, when the first *Atlas of Bronchioalveolar Lavage* was published by the German pneumologist Ulrich Costabel (2).

According to Costabel, Reynolds and Newball were the first clinicians who applied BAL in clinical routines in humans (3), not knowing that the method would become an accepted and broadly used diagnostic procedure recommended in internationally accepted guidelines (4).

Today, BALF is used for several diagnostic analyses including protein analyses in clinical chemistry, staining, and microscopy as well as flow cytometry and differential cell typing in pathology and cytology, and pathogen detection in microbiology and virology. Therefore, it is crucial to plan in advance which analyses are relevant for the respective clinical case and which BALF fractions should be used for which analyses.

The first step in the analysis of BALFs is processing for the differential cytology. While the individual procedures may vary among different

DOI: 10.1201/9781003146834-2

Table 1.1 Hematoxylin-eosin staining

Step	Reagent	Incubation time
1.	Hematoxylin	2 min.
2.	Running tap water	30 sec.
3.	Erythrosine B 1%	1 min.
4.	Running tap water	30 sec.
5.	Ethanol 75%	30 sec.
6.	Ethanol 96%	30 sec.
7.	Ethanol 100%	30 sec.
8.	Ethanol 100%	30 sec.
9.	Xylol	30 sec.
10.	Covering	

Reagents
- Mayer's Hematoxylin Solution, Sigma-Aldrich (Merck), Taufkirchen, Germany
- Erythorsin B dissolved in water, 1% (w/v), Sigma-Aldrich (Merck), Taufkirchen, Germany
- Covering medium, CV Mount, Leica, Wetzlar, Germany

laboratories, it has become an accepted strategy to filter the BALF through medical gauze in order to remove mucus and to enable a proper subsequent cytocentrifugation, usually for 5 minutes at 100 to 250 rpm depending on the type of rotor and centrifuge.

Subsequently, the resulting cytoslides are stained with common standard dyes used for cytology and histology like the May–Grünwald–Giemsa stain, hematoxylin-eosin stain, periodic acid–Schiff reaction, Prussian blue or Turnbull staining, and the Grocott-silver staining if fungi are suspected (4). An additional relevant staining in BAL cytology is Sudan Red–Hematoxylin fat staining, which is relevant in the case of aspiration pneumonia (5) and in cases of antiarrhythmic therapy with Amiodarone if lung toxic side effects occur (6–8). Detailed staining protocols are presented at the end of this chapter (Tables 1.1–1.6).

The cytological profile is the first and most important step to enable a sufficiently proper diagnosis, as the cytological profiles are characteristic for the different lung diseases.

Figure 1.1 gives an overview on the most frequently observed diseases with associated typical cell patterns detected in BALF that have been diagnosed between the years 2012 to 2022 in the Institute of Pathology, Hospital of the City of Cologne. These diseases were chronic eosinophilic pneumonia (CEP), eosinophilic granulomatosis with polyangiitis (EGPA), extrinsic allergic alveolitis (EAA), idiopathic pulmonary fibrosis (IPF), cryptogenic organizing pneumonia (COP), lung involvement in polymyositis, microscopic polyangiitis (MPA), sarcoidosis, sarcoidosis with neutrophilia, and *Pneumocystis jirovecii* pneumonia (PCP).

Table 1.2 May–Grünwald–Giemsa stain (MGG)

Step	Reagent	Time	Remarks
1.	May–Grünwald stain	30 sec.	
2.	Running tap water	30 sec.	Until water remains clear
3.	Giemsa Lösung 10%	30 min.	
4.	Running tap water	30 sec.	Until water remains clear
5.	Air dry		
6.	Xylol		
7.	Covering		

Reagents
- Buffer tablet pH6.8 preparing buffer solution acc. to WEISE for the staining of blood smears, Sigma-Aldrich (Merck), Taufkirchen, Germany for preparing a buffer (one tablet in 1,000 ml water)
- May–Grünwald stain, Sigma-Aldrich (Merck), Taufkirchen, Germany
- Giemsa-solution, Sigma-Aldrich (Merck), Taufkirchen, Germany; ready to use: 10% in buffer pH6.8 (v/v)
- Covering medium, CV Mount, Leica, Wetzlar, Germany

Table 1.3 Periodic acid–Schiff (PAS) staining

Step	Reagent	Time
1.	Incubation of slides at 84°C	20 min.
2.	Xylol	1 min.
3.	Xylol	1 min.
4.	Xylol	1 min.
5.	Ethanol 100%	1 min.
6.	Ethanol 96%	1 min.
7.	Ethanol 75%	1 min.
8.	Water	1 min.
9.	Periodic acid	1 min.
10.	Periodic acid	1 min.
11.	Distilled water	1 min.
12.	Distilled water	1 min.
13.	Schiff's reagent	1 min.
14.	Schiff's reagent	1 min.
15.	Schiff's reagent	1 min.
16.	Schiff's reagent	1 min.
17.	Running tap water	1 min.
18.	Running tap water	1 min.
19.	Hematoxylin	1 min.
20.	Hematoxylin	1 min.
21.	Hematoxylin	1 min.
22.	Running tap water	1 min.
23.	Running tap water	1 min.
24.	Ethanol 75%	1 min.
25.	Ethanol 96%	1 min.
26.	Ethanol 100%	1 min.
27.	Ethanol 100%	1 min.
28.	Xylol	
29.	Covering	

Reagents
- 1% periodic acid (w/v), Sigma-Aldrich (Merck), Taufkirchen, Germany
- Schiff's reagent, BioGnost, Zagreb, Croatia
- Covering medium, CV Mount, Leica, Wetzlar, Germany

Table 1.4 Prussian blue staining

Step	Reagent	Time
1.	Slide incubation at 84°C	20 min.
2.	Xylol	10 min.
3.	Xylol	10 min.
4.	Ethanol 100%	1 min.
5.	Ethanol 96%	1 min.
6.	Ethanol 75%	1 min.
7.	Aqua dest	1 min.
8.	10% potassium ferric hexacyanoferrate	10 min.
9.	Aqua dest	1min.
10.	Nuclear fast red	10 min.
11.	Tap water	1 min.
12.	Ethanol 75%	1 min.
13.	Ethanol 96%	1 min.
14.	Ethanol 100%	1 min.
15.	Xylol	1 min.
16.	Xylol	1 min.
17.	Covering	

Reagents
- Potassium-hexacyanoferrat(II)-Trihydrate, 60 ml 10% (w/v) plus 20 ml 10% hydrochloric acid, Sigma-Aldrich (Merck), Taufkirchen, Germany
- Nucleic Fast Red, 0.1%, Süsse Labortechnik, Gudensberg, Germany
- Covering medium, CV Mount, Leica, Wetzlar, Germany

Due to the fact that the diagnostic analysis of BALF is a sophisticated procedure, it requires considerable expertise in the laboratory as well as in the clinical setting. For this reason, this chapter is intended to provide a short introduction to this complex diagnostic field, whereas the following chapters, written by experts in their respective fields, focus on individual aspects in the context of relevant applications and clinical conditions to deliver the highest possible benefit for the readers.

Table 1.5 Silver staining

Step	Reagent	Time
1.	Slide incubation at 84°C	20 min.
2.	Xylol	10 min.
3.	Ethanol 100%	2 min.
4.	Ethanol 96%	2 min.
5.	Ethanol 75%	2 min.
6.	Potassium permanganate 1%	1 min.
7.	Tap water	short
8.	Potassium disulfite 2%	1 min.
9.	Tap water	short
10.	Ammonium iron(III) sulfate 2%	1 min.
11.	Tap water	short
12.	Distilled water	short
13.	Distilled water	short
14.	Ammoniacal silver nitrate solution	1 min.
15.	Distilled water	short
16.	Distilled water	short
17.	Formalin	1 min.
18.	Tap water	short
19.	Gold chloride 0.1%	10–20 min.
20.	Distilled water	short
21.	Potassium disulfite 2%	1 min.
22.	Tap water	short
23.	Sodium thiosulfate 1%	1 min.
24.	Tap water	short
25.	75% Ethanol	2 min.
26.	96% Ethanol	2 min.
27.	100% Ethanol	2 min.
28.	Xylol	2 min.
29.	CV Mount Leica	

Reagents

Potassium permanganate 1% (w/v), Sigma-Aldrich (Merck), Taufkirchen, Germany

Potassium disulfite 2% (w/v), Sigma-Aldrich (Merck), Taufkirchen, Germany

Ammonium iron(III) sulfate 2% (w/v), Sigma-Aldrich (Merck), Taufkirchen, Germany

Silver nitrate 10% (w/v), Sigma-Aldrich (Merck), Taufkirchen, Germany; 20 ml 10% silver nitrate (in water) were mixed with 4 ml potassium hydroxide solution (10% w/v); 25% of ammonium sulfate solution is added (dropwise) until silver nitrate is fully solved, then silver nitrate is added until the solution is saturated

Gold chloride solution, Süsse Labortechnik, Gudensberg, Germany

Sodium-thiosulfate-5-hydrate 1% (w/v), Sigma-Aldrich (Merck), Taufkirchen, Germany

Table 1.6 Sudan-II-fat staining

Step	Reagent	Time	Remarks
1.	Ethanol 50%	2–5 min.	
2.	Sudan-II solution	15–20 min.	
3.	Ethanol 50%	short	
4.	Distilled water	short	
5.	Hematoxylin	5–10 min.	
6.	Tap water	10 min.	
7.	Cover with Aquatex		

Reagents

- Mayer's Hematoxylin solution, Sigma-Aldrich (Merck), Taufkirchen, Germany
- Sudan-III solution: 0.2 to 0.3 g Sudan-III (Sigma-Aldrich (Merck), Taufkirchen, Germany) has to be dissolved in hot 70% ethanol and incubated at 37°C overnight. Let solution cool down to room temperature before usage and filter in advance. Addition of 6 ml water increases the staining power
- Aquatex, Sigma-Aldrich (Merck), Taufkirchen, Germany

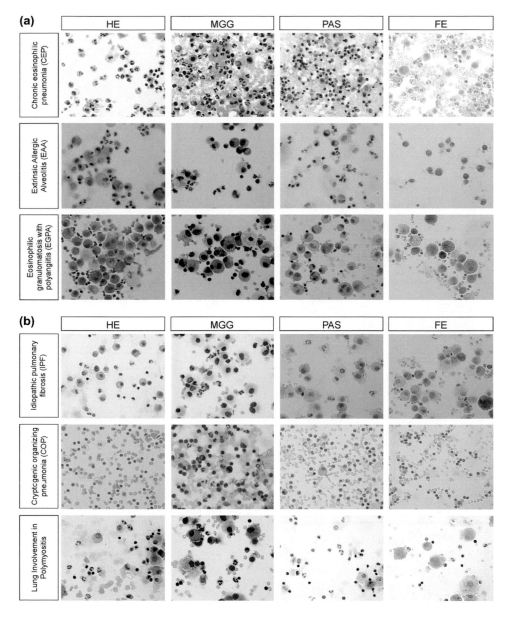

Figure 1.1 Overview of cytological staining of BALF cells found in the most frequently diagnosed diseases in the Institute of Pathology, Hospital of the City of Cologne, between 2012 and 2022.

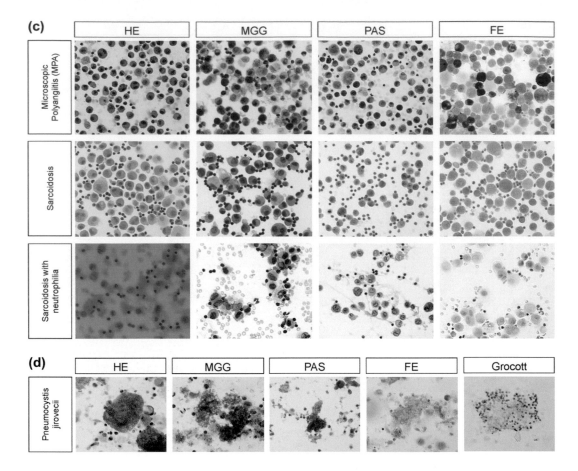

Figure 1.1 Continued

REFERENCES

1. Trobridge GF. Bronchial lavage. *Lancet.* 1957;272(6968):562–3.
2. Costabel U. *Atlas der bronchoalveolären Lavage.* Stuttgart, New York: Thieme; 1994. 99p.
3. Reynolds HY, Newball HH. Analysis of proteins and respiratory cells obtained from human lungs by bronchial lavage. *The Journal of Laboratory and Clinical Medicine.* 1974;84(4):559–73.
4. Meyer KC, Raghu G, Baughman RP, Brown KK, Costabel U, du Bois RM, et al. An official American Thoracic Society clinical practice guideline: The clinical utility of bronchoalveolar lavage cellular analysis in interstitial lung disease. *American Journal of Respiratory and Critical Care Medicine.* 2012;185(9):1004–14.
5. Mandell LA, Niederman MS. Aspiration pneumonia. *The New England Journal of Medicine.* 2019;380(7):651–63.
6. Papiris SA, Triantafillidou C, Kolilekas L, Markoulaki D, Manali ED. Amiodarone: Review of pulmonary effects and toxicity. *Drug Safety.* 2010;33(7):539–58.
7. Skeoch S, Weatherley N, Swift AJ, Oldroyd A, Johns C, Hayton C, et al. Drug-induced interstitial lung disease: A systematic review. *Journal of Clinical Medicine.* 2018;7(10).
8. Feduska ET, Thoma BN, Torjman MC, Goldhammer JE. Acute amiodarone pulmonary toxicity. *Journal of Cardiothoracic and Vascular Anesthesia.* 2021;35(5):1485–94.

2

Technical aspects of performing BAL

MIRIANA D'ALESSANDRO AND LAURA BERGANTINI

Bronchoalveolar lavage (BAL) is a non-invasive technique, and it is the simplest bronchoscopic procedure [1]. BAL was first performed in animal studies in 1961, aiming to harvest alveolar macrophages for research purposes [2]. Three years later, this method was introduced in humans.

A very interesting manuscript addressed the important issue of standardization: the European Society of Pneumology (SEP), in 1988, set up a Task Force on Bronchoalveolar Lavage [3]. The first report of the group focused specifically on technical recommendations and guidelines on how to perform BAL and how to process BAL material and was published in 1989 in the *ERJ* [3]. More recently, other recommendations from the BAL international task force have been developed from European Respiratory Society BAL Task Force Group guidelines [4].

Two different techniques to obtain a BAL during bronchoscopy procedure have been identified: low-pressure wall suction through a trap versus low pressure generated by a handheld syringe [5].

One of the main advantages of BAL is that it can be done as a daycare procedure [6]. A BAL procedure could discriminate between healthy and diseased tissue, and it is included in the diagnostic work-up of interstitial lung disease (ILD) [7].

Literature data that pertain to the performance of BAL document the considerable variability in technical aspects of performing BAL [8]. This may in part be the reason for apparent reluctance among pulmonologists worldwide to subject patients to BAL in the diagnostic evaluation of patients with ILD [9]. Several features affect the results of BAL cellular abnormalities. An underlying disease process or smoking may affect BAL bronchoscopy technique or analysis in several ways [10]. Airway obstruction leads to changes in BAL fluid return. This is due to the mechanical problem of aspirating fluid through narrowed airways that collapse when negative pressure is applied to facilitate fluid retrieval. In patients with chronic obstructive lung disease, the airway collapse is variable: the greater the negative pressure used to aspirate the fluid, significant airway collapse is more likely to occur and adversely influence the BAL fluid return [11]. In this regard, forced expiratory volume in the first second (FEV-1)/forced vital capacity (FVC) ratio has been correlated with the yield of BAL fluid return, the lower the ratio, the lower the proportion of BAL return.

Several features could affect the BAL performance. First of all, the position of the patient and the gravity that may impede lavage return from more gravity-dependent lung regions. Secondly, the choice of the most appropriate area or areas of the lungs for lavage. Since the 1970s, a main focus of research has been to investigate immune and inflammatory mechanisms in idiopathic pulmonary fibrosis (IPF) because of the especially poor prognosis and lack of effective therapies [12–15]. However, in the 1970s and 1980s several reports of BAL studies in the main groups of ILDs showed that differential BAL cell count findings were very similar from different centers using the right middle lobe or the right lower lobe as their standard lavage site [16]. In recent years, the use of high-resolution computed tomography (HRCT) and the importance of HRCT patterns in the new classification of idiopathic interstitial pneumonias, raises the possibility that differences in HRCT patterns in the lungs of individual patients may prove useful to identify target areas for BAL that may more accurately reflect the inflammatory cell profile that is associated with a specific ILD [17]. Further research is needed to better clarify whether different HRCT patterns are associated with different BAL cell profiles in the same lung and whether this would lead to major differences in the diagnostic interpretation compared with the current approach to using a standardized lavage site.

Generally, only one geographic area (lung segment) is lavaged when evaluating ILD. If multiple areas are lavaged, the specific lung regions that are lavaged should be noted.

Among the features affecting BAL performance, it has been to take into account the suction pressure during the procedure because of the airways' collapse when it is too high [18]. The majority of physicians in one survey used low-pressure wall suction (<60 mm Hg).

Finally, the total volume of normal saline instilled, the number of aliquots, and the volume of saline instilled in each aliquot for BAL. The major changes for both the cellular and protein contents of the BAL sample seem to occur during the first 100 ml of the process. The fluid aspirated after 60 ml instilled is significantly different than that obtained after 120 ml has been instilled. After two aliquots of 60 ml have been instilled and aspirated, the cells and protein returns appear to become consistent. Although some experts have suggested a specific number of aliquots be used

for BAL, there is considerable variability in the number and volume of aliquots used by pulmonologists. The choice of aliquot size on one side can easily be standardized as it is often determined by the size of the syringes available to the bronchoscopist in the local facility. On the other side, the European Respiratory Society recommends larger total instilled volumes of a minimum of 100 ml and a standard 240 ml using standard 4 × 60 ml aliquots to improve standardization when more efficient alveolar sampling and accurate quantitative measurements are required [19].

A minimal volume of 5 ml (optimal volume 10–20 ml) of a pooled BAL sample is recommended for BAL cellular analysis (the rest of the sample should be used for microbiology, virology, and malignant cell cytology laboratory testing as clinically indicated). BAL specimens should be collected in containers/aliquots that do not promote cell adherence to container surfaces. BAL specimens can be transported fresh at room temperature within 30 minutes following the collection, otherwise, they should be transported at 4°C (e.g., on ice) and delivered within 1 hour.

In the clinical routine laboratory, BAL is processed for cellular analysis (Figure 2.1) as follows: BAL is filtered through sterile gauze and cell count is determined by cytocentrifuge smear (600 rpm for 5 min) with a Thermo Shandon Cytospin 3 (Marshall Scientific, NH, USA), and stained with Diff-Quik stain kit (DiaPath, Italy); a total of 500 cells is counted. Cell viability is determined by Trypan blue exclusion in a Burker Chamber.

For BAL processing it is important that laboratories follow standard staining and processing methods. BAL fluid collected from bronchoscopy must be processed as soon as possible, in order to preserve the quality of samples and cell viability.

In order to maintain the viability of the samples, prior to processing the specimen needs to be kept at 4°C. Before starting the procedure, the samples need to be vortexed for 1 minute and then filtered through sterile gauze in order to remove mucus plugs. After vortexing, the samples will be transferred into a 50 ml tube using a serological pipette. If the BAL fluid appears turbid or contaminated by filaments, the fluid must be filtered through a 70 μm nylon mesh into a new 50 ml tube [20]. The following procedure will be carried out under sterile conditions in a biological safety

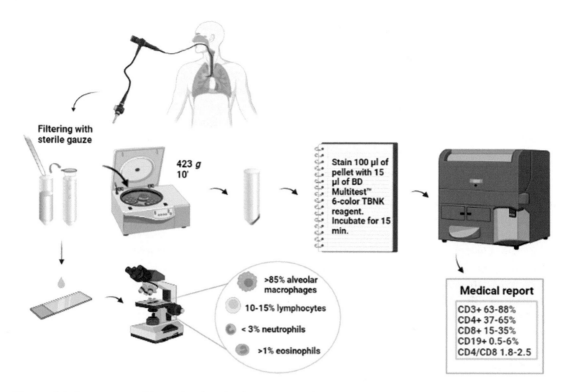

Figure 2.1 Processing of bronchoalveolar lavage samples.

cabinet, class II (BSL2) or higher. Generally, two applications are the most commonly used for BAL evaluation: microbiological analysis and cytological studies. In this chapter, we explain the cytological analysis.

CYTOLOGICAL ANALYSIS AND IMMUNE PHENOTYPING

Slides performance

Based on the density of cells, two or three droplets will be used to perform the slides. The centrifugation through cytocentrifuge for 10 minutes at 150 xg with cytospin will be used for the slides. Following the centrifugation, different stains can be applied based on the clinical evaluation.

Non-microbiological staining and interpretation

A variety of stains may be used in the interpretation of BAL specimens for different diagnostic purposes. The May–Grünwald–Giemsa is the

standard technique, useful for differential BAL cell count. A modified May–Grünwald–Giemsa stain, known as Diff-Quik, is a commonly used stain for cellular morphology [21]. Diff-Quik stain is very similar to traditional May–Grünwald stain, but it requires a considerably shortened staining time. Although these techniques are very similar, some differences appeared in cellular differential. In fact, Diff-Quik does not stain mast cells. These cells normally represent less than 1% of the usual nucleated cells in the BAL fluid, however they can provide clinical information related to specific lung disorders [22].

Regarding cellular subsets, it is also important to evidence that macrophages and lymphocytes can vary in size and shape, or they can appear as a single cell or in groups and/or clusters. The high degree of variability of these cells can lead to misidentification and misdiagnosis. Furthermore, macrophage cells may appear similar to lymphocytes and may be misinterpreted as intermediate or immature lymphocytes resulting in an increased lymphocyte count, or even lymphocytosis. A population of relatively young macrophages can be seen that are similar to lymphocytes. On the contrary, activated lymphocytes resulted in larger than steady-state lymphocytes and were mistaken for macrophages [23].

Macrophages can also appear as multinucleated cells and sometimes appear as full of granules. This phenomenon can be present in a variety of conditions including a history of smoking or mycobacteriosis. The nature of these granules can be identified through different stains. Carbon-based particles are the most common type of granules present in smokers or ex-smokers and are often present in alveolar macrophages that in this condition appear hyperchromatic [24].

For the identification of lipid-laden granules in macrophages in BAL cytology samples, the Oil red O stain is applied in the work-up of a number of clinical conditions, most notably for pulmonary aspiration. Oil red O stains lipid materials and imparts a red-orange color to the lipid and adipocytes and to visualize fat droplets or vacuoles.

However, different data suggested controversies in the use of this stain such as macrophage pigmentation, air bubble formation, and specimen cellularity. Recently it described the significance of this stain in diagnosing E-cigarette or vaping product use associated with lung injury [25].

Periodic acid–Schiff (PAS) staining is also used for the detection of structures that contain high concentrations of carbohydrate macromolecules (e.g., glycogen, glycoprotein, proteoglycan) typically found in connective tissue, mucus, and basal laminae. In BAL, PAS staining is mostly used to diagnose alveolar proteinosis [26].

Perls Prussian blue (PPB) stain recognizes Fe^{3+} associated with hemosiderin. Ferruginous bodies are intracellular structures, phagocytosed by lung macrophages. These are described as iron- and hemosiderin-laden macrophages and called either siderophages or sidero-macrophages and are associated with different pulmonary and extrapulmonary diseases [27].

Eosinophils and neutrophils can be also mistaken for one another. Increased eosinophils in the BAL occur in a limited number of conditions; however, with this information it is possible to make a diagnosis of eosinophilic pneumonia or associated conditions [28]. Eosinophil is most often bi-lobed, large, and round and has a typical aranciophile cytoplasm [29], while neutrophils may contain variable numbered nuclear lobes. If the morphologic character of the eosinophil is atypical (for example after degranulation processes) the better stain to distinguish them from the segmented neutrophil is the Papanicolaou stain [30].

Isolation and collection of supernatant

The samples will be centrifuged at 400 xg for 10 min at 4°C. Transfer the supernatant to a new 50 ml tube. Transfer 1.5 ml of the supernatant to each of 10 × 2 ml microcentrifuge tubes and the remaining supernatant to 15 ml tubes. Store all supernatant tubes at −80°C for 2 years or at −20°C for 6 months. Moreover, it is also important to evaluate what kind of molecules are to be tested in the study: some cytokines or chemokines, in fact, are susceptible to low temperatures.

Isolation and collection of cell pellet

Resuspend the pellet in 10 ml of RPMI 1640 for each 25 ml of the original collected samples. Centrifuge at 400 xg for 10 min at 4°C and then transfer the supernatant to a new 15 ml tube. Resuspend the pellet in 1 ml of RPMI 1640 + 10% fetal bovine serum (FBS) and count using Trypan blue and/or a hemocytometer if available. The cell pellet is considered good if the viability is greater than 90–95%. One million cells can be used for lymphocytes immunophenotyping that is described below. The resting cells can be collected in a cryovial after centrifugation at 300 xg for 10 min at 4°C [31]. Remove the supernatant and resuspend in 1.5 ml of freeze media in a cryogenic vial containing RPMI 1640 with 10% FBS and 10% of dimethyl sulfoxide (DMSO). Transfer the cryogenic vials to a controlled-rate freezing container and place them at −80°C. Transfer the cells to liquid nitrogen for long-term storage once the temperature is reached [20].

Lymphocytes immunophenotyping

Lymphocytes immunophenotyping is a routine test able to discriminate the principal subsets of lymphocytes. The test is performed through flow cytometry. One million cells were resuspended with 100 μl of specific buffer and 20 μl of monoclonal antibodies cocktail (BD Multitest™ 6-color TBNK, San Jose, CA, USA), including FITC-labeled CD3, PE-labeled CD16 and CD56, PerCP-Cy5.5-labeled CD45, PE-Cy7-labeled CD4, APC-labeled CD19, and APC-Cy7-labeled CD8 [32, 33]. The cell stained

for 30 minutes at room temperature. Centrifugation is performed for 10 minutes at 300 xg. Multitest™ 6-color TBNK is used to identify lymphocytes, which are distinguished on the basis of forward (FSC) versus side (SSC) scatters. Additional gating is applied using SSC versus CD45 to distinguish lymphocytes from cell debris. Specific panels are subsequently assessed to identify T lymphocytes, B lymphocytes, and NK cells. T lymphocyte sub-populations are gated in order to distinguish CD3+ CD4+ (T-helper), CD3+ CD8+ (T-cytotoxic), and CD3+ CD16/56+ cells (Figure 2.2).

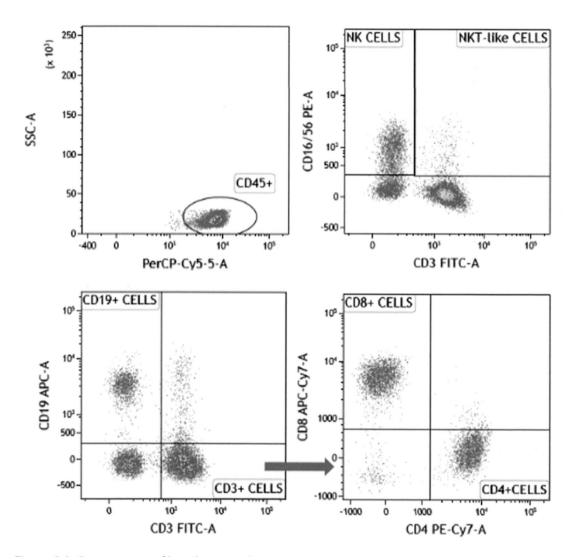

Figure 2.2 Gate strategy of lymphocyte subsets.

REFERENCES

1. K. R. Davidson, D. M. Ha, M. I. Schwarz, and E. D. Chan, *J Thorac Dis* 12(9), 4991 (2020).
2. J. Hetzel, M. Kreuter, C. M. Kähler, H. J. Kabitz, A. Gschwendtner, R. Eberhardt, U. Costabel, and K. Darwiche, *Sarcoidosis Vasc Diffuse Lung Dis* 38, e2021003 (2021).
3. U. Costabel, C. Danel, P. Haslam, T. Higgenbottam, H. Klech, W. Pohl, S. Rennard, G. Rossi, M. Rust, and G. Semenzato, *Eur Respir J* 2, 561 (1989).
4. P. L. Haslam and R. P. Baughman, *Eur Respir J* 14(2), 245 (1999).
5. C. Rosas-Salazar, S. A. Walczak, D. G. Winger, G. Kurland, and J. E. Spahr, *Pediatr Pulmonol* 49(10), 978 (2014).
6. S. Radha, T. Afroz, S. Prasad, and N. Ravindra, *J Cytol* 31(3), 136 (2014).
7. B. Efared, G. Ebang-Atsame, S. Rabiou, A. S. Diarra, L. Tahiri, N. Hammas, M. Smahi, B. Amara, M. C. Benjelloun, M. Serraj, L. Chbani, and H. El Fatemi, *J Negat Results Biomed* 16(1), 4 (2017).
8. D. B. Ettensohn, M. J. Jankowski, P. G. Duncan, and P. A. Lalor, *Chest* 94(2), 275 (1988).
9. L. Bergantini, M. d'Alessandro, P. Cameli, A. Perrone, B. Cekorja, B. Boncompagni, M. A. Mazzei, P. Sestini, and E. Bargagli, *Eur J Intern Med* 89, 76 (2021).
10. E. Bargagli, P. Cameli, A. Carleo, R. M. Refini, L. Bergantini, M. D'alessandro, L. Vietri, F. Perillo, L. Volterrani, P. Rottoli, L. Bini, and C. Landi, *Panminerva Med* 62(2), 109–115(2019).
11. M. S. Varegg, K. M. Kløverød, M. K. Austnes, N. Siwinska, M. Slowikowska, A. Zak, and A. Niedzwiedz, *J Vet Intern Med* 33(2), 976 (2019).
12. B. D. Bringardner, C. P. Baran, T. D. Eubank, and C. B. Marsh, *Antioxid Redox Signal* 10, 287 (2008).
13. N. W. Todd, I. G. Luzina, and S. P. Atamas, *Fibrogenesis Tissue Repair* 5(1), 11 (2012).
14. M. d'Alessandro, L. Bergantini, P. Cameli, M. Fanetti, L. Alderighi, M. Armati, R. M. Refini, V. Alonzi, P. Sestini, and E. Bargagli, *Int Immunopharmacol* 95, 107525 (2021).
15. M. d'Alessandro, L. Bergantini, P. Cameli, M. Pieroni, R. M. Refini, P. Sestini, and E. Bargagli, *Cancers (Basel)* 13(4), 689 (2021).
16. M. Heron, J. C. Grutters, K. M. ten Dam-Molenkamp, D. Hijdra, A. van Heugten-Roeling, A. M. E. Claessen, H. J. T. Ruven, J. M. M. van den Bosch, and H. van Velzen-Blad, *Clin Exp Immunol* 167(3), 523 (2012).
17. M. T. A. Buzan and C. M. Pop, *Clujul Med* 88(2), 116 (2015).
18. K. Singh, S. Khan, S. Agarwal, G. Walters, and E. E. McGrath, *Ann Thorac Surg* 97(2), 720 (2014).
19. S. R. Zaidi, A. M. Collins, E. Mitsi, J. Reiné, K. Davies, A. D. Wright, J. Owugha, R. Fitzgerald, A. Ganguli, S. B. Gordon, D. M. Ferreira, and J. Rylance, *BMC Pulm Med* 17(1), 83 (2017).
20. K. C. Meyer, G. Raghu, R. P. Baughman, K. K. Brown, U. Costabel, R. M. du Bois, M. Drent, P. L. Haslam, D. S. Kim, S. Nagai, P. Rottoli, C. Saltini, M. Selman, C. Strange, B. Wood, and American Thoracic Society Committee on BAL in Interstitial Lung Disease, *Am J Respir Crit Care Med* 185(9), 1004 (2012).
21. K. K. Woronzoff-Dashkoff, *Clin Lab Med* 22(1), 15 (2002).
22. F. Stanzel, in *Principles and Practice of Interventional Pulmonology*, edited by A. Ernst and F. J. Herth (Springer, New York, 2013), pp. 165–176.
23. G. Rossi, A. Cavazza, P. Spagnolo, S. Bellafiore, E. Kuhn, P. Carassai, L. Caramanico, G. Montanari, G. Cappiello, A. Andreani, F. Bono, and N. Nannini, *Eur Respir Rev* 26(145), 170009 (2017).
24. J. L. Pauly, S. J. Stegmeier, A. G. Mayer, J. D. Lesses, and R. J. Streck, *Tob Control* 6(1), 33 (1997).
25. S. Niu, G. R. Colon, K. Molberg, H. Chen, K. Carrick, S. Yan, V. Sarode, and E. Lucas, *Diagn Cytopathol* 49(7), 876 (2021).
26. H. P. Hauber and P. Zabel, *Diagn Pathol* 4, 13 (2009).
27. A. J. Ghio and V. L. Roggli, *J Environ Pathol Toxicol Oncol* 40(1), 1 (2021).

28. P. Paul, P. Patel, S. K. Verma, P. Mishra, B. R. Sahu, P. K. Panda, G. S. Kushwaha, S. Senapati, N. Misra, and M. Suar, *Cell Biol Toxicol* 38(1), 111 (2022).

29. B. M. Skinner and E. E. P. Johnson, *Chromosoma* 126(2), 195 (2017).

30. L. George and C. E. Brightling, *Ther Adv Chronic Dis* 7(1), 34 (2016).

31. N. Kneidinger, J. Warszawska, P. Schenk, V. Fuhrmann, A. Bojic, A. Hirschl, H. Herkner, C. Madl, and A. Makristathis, *Crit Care* 17(4), R135 (2013).

32. I. F. de M. Picinin, P. Camargos, R. F. Mascarenhas, S. M. E. Santos, and C. Marguet, *Eur Respir J* 38(3), 738 (2011).

33. R. J. Harbeck, *Clin Diagn Lab Immunol* 5(3), 271 (1998).

3

BAL as a research tool

MIRIANA D'ALESSANDRO AND ELENA BARGAGLI

Bronchoalveolar lavage (BAL) is essential in the diagnostic algorithm of pulmonary diseases to better define diagnosis including in tuberculosis, fungal infections, bacterial pneumonias, and malignancies [1–4]. BAL performed during bronchoscopy has diagnostic indication for interstitial lung diseases (ILDs) including sarcoidosis, eosinophilic pneumonia, and pulmonary Langerhans cell histiocytosis [5]. BAL can allow a specific diagnosis, or it can contribute to the differential diagnosis between different lung diseases [6–8].

BAL is also a perfect matrix to better define disease activity and to study the pathogenesis of many diseases through its cellular composition analysis and lymphocyte phenotyping [5, 9–13].

The actual value of a BAL is to rule out granulomatous infections such as fungal or mycobacterial infection. The BAL should be performed before any biopsy attempt to avoid blood contamination [14].

Different methodologies have been applied to the study of BAL to identify pathogenetic mechanisms of lung diseases, including OMICs (The branches of science known informally as omics are various disciplines in biology whose names end in the suffix -omics, such as genomics, proteomics) [15].

Since BAL proteome directly reflects lung physiology and pathology better than plasma proteome, the former has been more widely applied in the study of ILD [16, 17]. Researchers have used different techniques in the study of various lung diseases by BAL in relation to their experimental design.

Notably, these proteomic tools provide a means to assess global changes in the composition of respiratory secretions in response to various inflammatory stimuli or in association with certain disease states [18]. Proteomic techniques have also been used to identify BAL fluid proteins in wild-type mice and in murine models of lung injury and disease [19].

For example, changes in sample preparation and electrophoretic separation have been made to improve the analysis of low molecular weight proteins and by these enriched samples interesting polypeptides were found in BAL of pulmonary alveolar proteinosis patients [20]. Although many studies on BAL proteomes are available, sample preparation is still a critical step in two-dimensional electrophoresis (2-DE), as indicated by a very interesting paper by Leroy [21]. BAL proteomic studies of protein patterns involved in the pathogenesis of idiopathic pulmonary fibrosis (IPF) to find potential biomarkers are of interest as well as the research studies focusing on the comparison between IPF and other ILDs and IPF patients compared with healthy smoker and non-smoker controls [22–25].

Cigarette smoking may influence BAL protein composition and is known as a potential

DOI: 10.1201/9781003146834-4

risk factor for interstitial lung diseases, especially IPF [25]. The association of tobacco smoke with impaired cell motility and wound healing is well documented [26, 27]. Tobacco smoke contains many toxic and carcinogenic compounds that interact with DNA, lipids, and proteins in different organs to alter their normal physiological activities, ultimately causing adverse health effects [28]. Cigarette smoke creates a field of molecular injury in the epithelial lining of the entire respiratory tract [29]. Changes include cell atypia, allelic loss, and promoter hypermethylation [30]. Exposure induces differential secretion of proteins associated with a variety of biological processes, including metabolic, regulatory, developmental, and signaling processes, as well as responses to stimulus and stress [31].

BAL fluid is a useful source of biomarkers, but it has some limitations to be considered for proteomic analysis: high salt concentrations, dilution of low Mw proteins, and abundance of plasma high Mw proteins, but they can be partially corrected by appropriate expedients according to the applied techniques (dialysis, concentration of the sample, removal of high Mw proteins, etc.) [32].

Nevertheless, the analysis of alveolar proteins could elucidate the pathogenesis of several lung diseases, including ILD [33, 34]. This is the case of transmembrane mucins that play a key role in the lung, and they are mainly implicated in the process of cellular proliferation, growth, and apoptosis, with increased expression in injured or regenerating epithelial cells (e.g., Krebs von den Lungen-6/MUC1, MUC4, and MUC16) [35]. There is growing interest in the investigation of the diagnostic and prognostic role of mucins in different lung diseases including ILD [36]. It further shines a spotlight on the role of transmembrane mucins in rheumatologic disorders associated with ILD and the unmet need to identify those patients with lung involvement, because of the inexorable worsening of patients when the concomitant interstitial lung involvement [37].

KL-6 is a high molecular weight (200 kDa) glycoprotein, firstly suggested as a serum biomarker for several types of cancer (although with low diagnostic accuracy) [36].

Immunohistochemical studies have shown that KL-6 is strongly expressed in Type 2 pneumocytes, though it has not been clarified whether the increased concentrations of KL-6 in sera from patients with ILD are exclusively derived from the lower respiratory tract [38].

The pathophysiologic role of epithelial mucins produced by Type 2 pneumocytes has not been fully clarified. The Type 2 pneumocytes, as multipotent progenitors, have a role in the repair of injured alveolar epithelium by covering the space where damaged Type 1 pneumocytes have desquamated from the basement membrane [39]. Since it has been demonstrated that activated Type 2 pneumocytes show increased production of TGF-beta in patients with IPF and TGF-beta is mitogenic for fibroblasts, Type 2 pneumocytes may be involved in the cellular and molecular pathways of fibrotic development [40].

To date, limited data are available for the comparison of alveolar and peripheral KL-6 concentrations in ILD patients, though it could reflect the damage in the lower respiratory tract of fibrotic patients and could have prognostic meaning, discriminating progressive and non-progressive patients [41].

Several authors reported lower KL-6 concentrations in BAL than the serum of fibrotic ILD patients compared to non-fibrotic [42]. This finding could be explained by the hypothesis that the irreversible damage in fibrotic ILD patients leads to KL-6 migration through the basal membrane to peripheral blood.

New flow cytometry (FCM) methods using fluorescence-encoded beads suitable for use on various flow cytometers has been employed to simultaneously quantify several soluble proteins.

Recent research has focused on the pathogenesis of various types of interstitial lung disorders where BAL supernatant and cell counts may further contribute to better define these conditions or to be of some clinical value to assess the differential diagnosis, activity of disease, and to provide prognostic information [43, 44]. D'Alessandro et al. investigated and compared the expression of different lipid mediators, including adipokines, in BAL and serum of IPF and fibrotic hypersensitivity pneumonitis (HP) patients [45]. The differential diagnosis between these two diseases is still challenging and the authors identified a BAL lipid biomarker panel to support the hypothesis that fibrotic HP and IPF have different lung fibrosis phenotypes: the former is a post-inflammatory cell-regulated ILD and the second is more related to tissue remodeling and repair.

There is increasing evidence that the analysis of biomarkers in BAL fluid samples could be helpful in clinical practice to elucidate the pathogenesis of several lung diseases, mainly ILD.

Over the last few years, there has been increasing evidence of the involvement of extracellular vesicles (EVs) in the pathogenesis of lung diseases, including lung cancer, chronic obstructive pulmonary disease, and pulmonary fibrosis [46–49]. It has been speculated that EVs play a pivotal role as mediators of cell–cell communication, as well as having a cooperator role in the development of lung diseases such as IPF [47, 50, 51].

EVs carry a wide variety of bioactive molecules such as DNA, RNA, lipids, and proteins, which enable them to regulate host cell activity and behavior by activating different signaling pathways [52]. However, the role of EVs and their translational applications in fibrotic ILD patients is relatively unexplored, despite their likely potential as diagnostic and theranostic markers of fibrotic ILDs [53].

Standardized recovery of EVs from an EV-containing matrix is still challenging and many questions remain about the effects of specific pre-analytical variables on different classes of EVs as well as their isolation techniques in BAL fluid samples from ILD patients is still a matter of debate.

Recently, FCM bead-based methods allow the definition of cytokine expression patterns by cell components of BAL samples, including lymphocyte tying. Monoclonal antibody combinations have been exploited to identify BAL leukocytes. However, there are no guidelines yet about approaching panels and gates strategies. A new profile of monoclonal antibodies allows the BAL leukocyte counting to identify lymphocytes such as CD15−, CD16−, and CD16^{dim} (NK lymphocytes), and HLA-DR− and HLA-DR+ (B cells and activated lymphocytes) cells; neutrophils such as CD15^{bright}, CD16^{bright}, HLA-DR− cells; eosinophils such as CD15^{bright}, CD16−, and HLA-DR− cells; and alveolar macrophages such as CD15^{dim}, CD16^{bright}, and HLA-DR^{bright} cells [54]. The macrophage's autofluorescence was overcome using the monoclonal antibody anti-HLA-DR conjugated with the dye allophycocyanin (APC) as the main identification marker.

Most studies of BAL were performed in sarcoidosis patients, probably due to the diagnostic purpose of bronchoscopy with BAL in the sarcoidosis diagnostic work-up. Despite the fact that sarcoidosis is still an idiopathic granulomatous disease, BAL samples from such patients showed CD4+ T cells highly Th1 polarized which is crucial for the inflammatory process in sarcoidosis [9, 55]. For this reason, a BAL cell pattern with a CD4/CD8 ratio of >3.5 has been postulated as a potential diagnostic indication of sarcoidosis [56].

Considering the infiltration of Th1-polarized CD4+ T cells in the lung, it is widely accepted that these T cells are trafficking to and proliferating in the lung in response to an unknown antigen [9]. In contrast to CD4+ T cell alveolitis in BAL of sarcoidosis patients, T cell lymphopenia in the peripheral blood is characteristic of the disease [57]. CD4+ T cells with a Th17 phenotype and T cells expressing both IL-17 and IFN-γ (i.e., Th17.1 cells) have been found in lung tissue and BAL from sarcoidosis [58]. Recently, it was demonstrated a significant increase in CCR6+ Th17.1 cells in both BAL fluid and mediastinal lymph nodes of sarcoidosis patients compared to controls [59]. Interestingly these cells contribute to IFN-γ production. It is believed that disturbance of Th17-stimulated regulatory T cells (Tregs) can lead to autoimmune inflammation, characterized by the presence of autoantigen-specific T and B lymphocytes producing autoantibodies [60]. Disturbances in T and B cell immune responses have been reported in several studies of sarcoidosis, suggesting that the triggering factor for inflammation is contact of a foreign antigen with antigen-presenting cells, leading to activation of T and B lymphocytes, which migrate to the inflammatory foci [61]. If the antigen persists, macrophages undergo epithelioid differentiation and lymphocytes continue to migrate to the foci, forming granulomas. B cell involvement in sarcoidosis is therefore well documented [62], but nothing is known about T follicular helper (Tfh) cells in this disease. Tfh is the major cell subset considered to be involved in humoral adaptive immune response, due to its essential role in generating plasma and memory B cells during germinal center reaction [63]. Tfh cells express high levels of the chemokine receptor CXCR5 necessary for Tfh migration towards B cell follicles rich in CXCL13 (B cell chemoattractant) [64]. Additionally, specific stimulation of Tfh cells induces secretion of IL-21, thereby promoting B cell growth, differentiation, and class-switching [65].

Recently, similarities with autoimmune diseases suggest that autoimmune components play an important role in the pathogenesis of sarcoidosis. D'Alessandro et al. demonstrated for the first time a link between imbalance in circulating and alveolar Tfh cells, especially CCR4-, CXCR3-, and CXCR5-expressing Tfh subsets, in the development of sarcoidosis [66]. These findings raise questions about the pathogenesis of sarcoidosis and may provide new directions for future clinical studies and treatment strategies.

Sarcoidosis is driven by a T cell mechanism, in particular accumulation of activated CD4+ T cells in the lungs, allowing T cell attachment and transmigration through the endothelium, endorsed by expression of integrins [67, 68]. Integrins are a large family of transmembrane proteins and the main receptors for extracellular matrix components. Most studies on CD4+ and CD8+ T cell subpopulations have identified an integrin alpha-E beta-7 (CD103), an adhesion molecule with αE and β7 subunits [69]. This molecule can promote T cell migration into the epithelium and is involved in retaining lymphocytes in the mucosa [70]. The literature on sarcoidosis reports CD103 to be stage-dependent, mainly related to stages II and III [71]. CD103 is certainly expressed on 95% of intraepithelial CD4+ lymphocytes in the mucosa, but on less than 2% of circulating peripheral blood lymphocytes [69]. Sarcoidosis patients show lower CD103 expression on BAL CD4+ cells than patients with other granulomatous ILDs, suggesting that these cells are of peripheral origin [6].

D'Alessandro et al. analyzed the different distribution and compartmentalization of CD103 expression on T cell subsets in BAL fluid, peripheral blood, and lymph node tissue from sarcoidosis patients [9].

They firstly reported a link between imbalance in circulating, alveolar, and lymph node CD8+ and CD8+CD103+ T cells, ThReg (CD4+CD25+CD127-), Tfh (CD4+CXCR5+), and ThNaïve (CD4+CD25-CD127+) and the CD103+CD4+/CD4+ T cell ratio in the development of sarcoidosis [9].

Additional testing in BAL the immune-checkpoint (IC) expression (such as programmed cell death-1, PD-1) on T cells has proven to be involved in the pathogenesis of sarcoidosis and is associated with computed tomography (CT) evidence of spontaneous improvement [72].

T cell activation is regulated by co-stimulatory factors, such as CD28, and co-inhibitory factors, such as IC molecules [73]. The suppression of T cells occurs during binding of the T cell receptor to antigen/major histocompatibility complex with the involvement of IC molecules. D'Alessandro et al. reported a detailed comparison of the expression of PD-1 and cytotoxic T lymphocyte antigen 4 (CTLA-4) as negative regulators of activated T cells, and the T cell immunoglobulin and ITIM domain (TIGIT) as the next generation of IC molecules which also suppressively regulate immune responses of T cells through their unique signals, in three different anatomical compartments side-by-side in the same patient in order to better elucidate the immune responses associated with the development and progression of sarcoidosis [74]. The authors revealed a high expression of PD1 and TIGIT on T cells in BAL, as well as CTLA-4 and TIGIT on T cells in lymph nodes, suggesting that inhibition of these molecules could be a therapeutic strategy for avoiding the development of chronic inflammation and tissue damage in sarcoidosis patients [74].

IC molecules are also overexpressed on NK cells, inducing cell exhaustion. NK and NKT-like (CD3+CD16+CD56+) cells are gradually becoming focal points in research efforts to unravel the pathways influencing granuloma resolution and persistence [75]. Bergantini et al. firstly reported the differently expression of such cells in BAL from patients with different ILD and were significantly depleted in sarcoidosis with respect to other ILDs [10]. The authors speculated a protective role of NK and NKT-like cells in the pathogenesis of sarcoidosis, and they suggested a cut-off value of 1.65% of NK cells in BAL as indicative marker for sarcoidosis diagnosis [10].

Moreover, the variations of NK cells in the BAL from 159 patients with distinct fibrotic ILD phenotypes were described suggesting a potential role for IPF prognosis and progression [76]. However, many questions remain unanswered, such as the immunomodulatory role of NKT cells on the important alveolar type 2 to alveolar type 1 cell transition during lung injury, the behavior of these cells in lung parenchyma as opposed to the alveolar spaces and the applicability of NKT-based immunotherapies on ILD, whose natural history, progression and prognosis is highly variable [77].

BAL is a useful biomarker resource for pathogenesis, diagnosis, and prognosis of lung diseases, including ILD. BAL is a biological matrix to better define disease activity and to study the pathogenesis of many diseases in order to translate such information into effective therapies into clinical practice as new therapeutic strategies.

REFERENCES

1. P. L. Haslam and R. P. Baughman, *Eur Respir J* 14(2), 245 (1999).
2. S.-P. Hogea, E. Tudorache, C. Pescaru, M. Marc, and C. Oancea, *Expert Rev Respir Med* 14(11), 1117 (2020).
3. K. C. Meyer, *Semin Respir Crit Care Med* 28(5), 546 (2007).
4. V. Poletti, G. Poletti, B. Murer, L. Saragoni, and M. Chilosi, *Semin Respir Crit Care Med* 28(5), 534 (2007).
5. K. C. Meyer, G. Raghu, R. P. Baughman, K. K. Brown, U. Costabel, R. M. du Bois, M. Drent, P. L. Haslam, D. S. Kim, S. Nagai, P. Rottoli, C. Saltini, M. Selman, C. Strange, B. Wood, and American Thoracic Society Committee on BAL in Interstitial Lung Disease, *Am J Respir Crit Care Med* 185(9), 1004 (2012).
6. M. d'Alessandro, A. Carleo, P. Cameli, L. Bergantini, A. Perrone, L. Vietri, N. Lanzarone, C. Vagaggini, P. Sestini, and E. Bargagli, *Clin Exp Med* 20(2), 207 (2020).
7. P. Rottoli and E. Bargagli, *Curr Opin Pulm Med* 9(5), 418 (2003).
8. K. C. Meyer and G. Raghu, *Eur Respir J* 38(4), 761 (2011).
9. M. d'Alessandro, S. Gangi, D. Cavallaro, L. Bergantini, F. Mezzasalma, S. Cattelan, S. Baglioni, M. Abbritti, P. Cameli, and E. Bargagli, *Life (Basel)* 12(5), 762 (2022).
10. L. Bergantini, P. Cameli, M. d'Alessandro, C. Vagaggini, R. M. Refini, C. Landi, M. G. Pieroni, M. Spalletti, P. Sestini, and E. Bargagli, *Clin Exp Med* 19(4), 487 (2019).
11. Y.-R. A. Yu, D. F. Hotten, Y. Malakhau, E. Volker, A. J. Ghio, P. W. Noble, M. Kraft, J. W. Hollingsworth, M. D. Gunn, and R. M. Tighe, *Am J Respir Cell Mol Biol* 54(1), 13 (2016).
12. S. Strippoli, L. Fucci, A. Negri, D. Putignano, M. L. Cisternino, G. Napoli, R. Filannino, I. De Risi, A. M. Sciacovelli, and M. Guida, *J Transl Med* 18(1), 473 (2020).
13. L. Barss, K. L. Fraser, M. M. Kelly, and K. A. Johannson, *Eur Respir J* 51(3), 1701769 (2018).
14. https://www.sciencedirect.com/topics/medicine-and-dentistry/lung-lavage.
15. G. Yu, G. H. Ibarra, and N. Kaminski, *Matrix Biol* 68–69, 422 (2018).
16. Q. K. Li, P. Shah, Y. Li, P. O. Aiyetan, J. Chen, R. Yung, D. Molena, E. Gabrielson, F. Askin, D. W. Chan, and H. Zhang, *J Proteome Res* 12(8), 3689 (2013).
17. J. Hirsch, K. C. Hansen, A. L. Burlingame, and M. A. Matthay, *Am J Physiol Lung Cell Mol Physiol* 287(1), L1 (2004).
18. J. A. Bartlett, M. E. Albertolle, C. Wohlford-Lenane, A. A. Pezzulo, J. Zabner, R. K. Niles, S. J. Fisher, P. B. McCray, and K. E. Williams, *Am J Physiol Lung Cell Mol Physiol* 305(3), L256 (2013).
19. C.-C. Chang, S.-H. Chen, S.-H. Ho, C.-Y. Yang, H.-D. Wang, and M.-L. Tsai, *Proteomics* 7(23), 4388 (2007).
20. X.-F. Xu, H.-P. Dai, Y.-M. Li, F. Xiao, and C. Wang, *Chin Med J (Engl)* 129(19), 2357 (2016).
21. B. Leroy, P. Falmagne, and R. Wattiez, *Methods Mol Biol* 425, 67 (2008).
22. E. Bargagli, R. M. Refini, M. d'Alessandro, L. Bergantini, P. Cameli, L. Vantaggiato, L. Bini, and C. Landi, *Int J Mol Sci* 21(16) (2020).

23. C. Landi, E. Bargagli, A. Carleo, L. Bianchi, A. Gagliardi, A. Prasse, M. G. Perari, R. M. Refini, L. Bini, and P. Rottoli, *Proteomics Clin Appl* 8(11–12), 932 (2014).

24. P. Cameli, A. Carleo, L. Bergantini, C. Landi, A. Prasse, and E. Bargagli, *Inflammation* 43(1), 1 (2020).

25. E. Bargagli, P. Cameli, A. Carleo, R. M. Refini, L. Bergantini, M. D'alessandro, L. Vietri, F. Perillo, L. Volterrani, P. Rottoli, L. Bini, and C. Landi, *Panminerva Med* 62(2), 109–115 (2019).

26. A. A. D. Lassig, J. E. Bechtold, B. R. Lindgren, A. Pisansky, A. Itabiyi, B. Yueh, and A. M. Joseph, *Laryngoscope* 128(3), 618 (2018).

27. Y. Fang and K. K. H. Svoboda, *J Clin Periodontol* 32(12), 1200 (2005).

28. National Center for Chronic Disease Prevention and Health, *Pulmonary Diseases* (Centers for Disease Control and Prevention (US), 2010).

29. K. Steiling, J. Ryan, J. S. Brody, and A. Spira, *Cancer Prev Res (Phila)* 1(6), 396 (2008).

30. S. M. Simet, J. H. Sisson, J. A. Pavlik, J. M. DeVasure, C. Boyer, X. Liu, S. Kawasaki, J. G. Sharp, S. I. Rennard, and T. A. Wyatt, *Am J Respir Cell Mol Biol* 43(6), 635 (2010).

31. G. S. Hotamisligil and R. J. Davis, *Cold Spring Harb Perspect Biol* 8(10), a006072 (2016).

32. A. Hmmier, M. E. O'Brien, V. Lynch, M. Clynes, R. Morgan, and P. Dowling, *BBA Clin* 7, 97 (2017).

33. J. A. Whitsett, S. E. Wert, and T. E. Weaver, *Annu Rev Med* 61, 105 (2010).

34. H. H. Popper, *Virchows Arch* 462(1), 1 (2013).

35. J. Ma, B. K. Rubin, and J. A. Voynow, *Chest* 154(1), 169 (2018).

36. M. d'Alessandro, L. Bergantini, P. Cameli, L. Vietri, N. Lanzarone, V. Alonzi, M. Pieroni, R. M. Refini, P. Sestini, F. Bonella, and E. Bargagli, *Biomark Med* 14(8), 665 (2020).

37. B. A. Symmes, A. L. Stefanski, C. M. Magin, and C. M. Evans, *Biochem Soc Trans* 46(3), 707 (2018).

38. N. Kohno, Y. Awaya, T. Oyama, M. Yamakido, M. Akiyama, Y. Inoue, A. Yokoyama, H. Hamada, S. Fujioka, and K. Hiwada, *Am Rev Respir Dis* 148(3), 637 (1993).

39. C. Zhao, X. Fang, D. Wang, F. Tang, and X. Wang, *Respir Med* 104(10), 1391 (2010).

40. K. K. Kim, D. Sheppard, and H. A. Chapman, *Cold Spring Harb Perspect Biol* 10(4), a022293 (2018).

41. Y. Jiang, Q. Luo, Q. Han, J. Huang, Y. Ou, M. Chen, Y. Wen, S. S. Mosha, K. Deng, and R. Chen, *J Thorac Dis* 10(8), 4705 (2018).

42. C. Chung, J. Kim, H. S. Cho, and H. C. Kim, *Sci Rep* 12(1), 8564 (2022).

43. U. Costabel and J. Guzman, *Curr Opin Pulm Med* 7(5), 255 (2001).

44. M. d'Alessandro, L. Bergantini, R. M. Refini, P. Cameli, F. Perillo, C. Landi, F. Icorne, A. Perrone, P. Sestini, F. Bonella, and E. Bargagli, *Immunobiology* 225(5), 151997 (2020).

45. M. d'Alessandro, L. Bergantini, P. Cameli, N. Lanzarone, F. Perillo, A. Perrone, and E. Bargagli, *Life Sci* 256, 117995 (2020).

46. T. Kadota, Y. Yoshioka, Y. Fujita, K. Kuwano, and T. Ochiya, *Semin Cell Dev Biol* 67, 39 (2017).

47. D. Chanda, E. Otoupalova, K. P. Hough, M. L. Locy, K. Bernard, J. S. Deshane, R. D. Sanderson, J. A. Mobley, and V. J. Thannickal, *Am J Respir Cell Mol Biol* 60(3), 279 (2019).

48. A. Martin-Medina, M. Lehmann, O. Burgy, S. Hermann, H. A. Baarsma, D. E. Wagner, M. M. De Santis, F. Ciolek, T. P. Hofer, M. Frankenberger, M. Aichler, M. Lindner, W. Gesierich, A. Guenther, A. Walch, C. Coughlan, P. Wolters, J. S. Lee, J. Behr, and M. Königshoff, *Am J Respir Crit Care Med* 198(12), 1527 (2018).

49. S. Sato, S. G. Chong, C. Upagupta, T. Yanagihara, T. Saito, C. Shimbori, P.-S. Bellaye, Y. Nishioka, and M. R. Kolb, *Thorax* 76(9), 895 (2021).

50. X. Wan, S. Chen, Y. Fang, W. Zuo, J. Cui, and S. Xie, *J Cell Physiol* 235(11), 8613 (2020).

51. M. d'Alessandro, P. Soccio, L. Bergantini, P. Cameli, G. Scioscia, M. P. Foschino Barbaro, D. Lacedonia, and E. Bargagli, *Cells* 10(5), 1045 (2021).
52. C. Théry, K. W. Witwer, E. Aikawa, M. J. Alcaraz, et al., *J Extracell Vesicles* 7(1), 1535750 (2018).
53. M. d'Alessandro, L. Bergantini, E. Bargagli, and S. Vidal, *Life (Basel)* 11(12), 1401 (2021).
54. L. Tricas, A. Echeverría, M. A. Blanco, M. Menéndez, and J. Belda, *Cytom B* 82(2), 61 (2012).
55. C. Agostini, A. Meneghin, and G. Semenzato, *Curr Opin Pulm Med* 8(5), 435 (2002).
56. U. Costabel and G. W. Hunninghake, *Eur Respir J* 14(4), 735 (1999).
57. J. Grunewald and A. Eklund, *Proc Am Thorac Soc* 4(5), 461 (2007).
58. J. Ramstein, C. E. Broos, L. J. Simpson, K. M. Ansel, S. A. Sun, M. E. Ho, P. G. Woodruff, N. R. Bhakta, L. Christian, C. P. Nguyen, B. J. Antalek, B. S. Benn, R. W. Hendriks, B. van den Blink, M. Kool, and L. L. Koth, *Am J Respir Crit Care Med* 193(11), 1281 (2016).
59. S. A. Greaves, S. M. Atif, and A. P. Fontenot, *Front Immunol* 11, 474 (2020).
60. A. Jäger and V. K. Kuchroo, *Scand J Immunol* 72(3), 173 (2010).
61. A. A. Starshinova, A. M. Malkova, N. Y. Basantsova, Y. S. Zinchenko, I. V. Kudryavtsev, G. A. Ershov, L. A. Soprun, V. A. Mayevskaya, L. P. Churilov, and P. K. Yablonskiy, *Front Immunol* 10, 2933 (2020).
62. I. Kudryavtsev, M. Serebriakova, A. Starshinova, Y. Zinchenko, N. Basantsova, A. Malkova, L. Soprun, L. P. Churilov, E. Toubi, P. Yablonskiy, and Y. Shoenfeld, *Sci Rep* 10(1), 1059 (2020).
63. D. Breitfeld, L. Ohl, E. Kremmer, J. Ellwart, F. Sallusto, M. Lipp, and R. Förster, *J Exp Med* 192(11), 1545 (2000).
64. D. A. Rao, *Front Immunol* 9, 1924 (2018).
65. R. I. Nurieva and Y. Chung, *Cell Mol Immunol* 7(3), 190 (2010).
66. M. d'Alessandro, L. Bergantini, P. Cameli, F. Mezzasalma, R. M. Refini, M. Pieroni, P. Sestini, and E. Bargagli, *Clin Exp Immunol* 205(3), 406 (2021).
67. M. Couto, C. Palmares, M. Beltrão, S. Neves, P. Mota, A. Morais, and L. Delgado, *Int Arch Occup Environ Health* 88(2), 167 (2015).
68. https://pubmed.ncbi.nlm.nih.gov /34232700/.
69. R. Aleksonienė, J. Besusparis, V. Gruslys, L. Jurgauskienė, A. Laurinavičienė, A. Laurinavičius, R. Malickaitė, J. Norkūnienė, R. Zablockis, E. Žurauskas, and E. Danila, *J Thorac Dis* 13(4), 2300 (2021).
70. J. Lohmeyer, J. Friedrich, F. Grimminger, U. Maus, R. Tenter, H. Morr, H. G. Velcovsky, W. Seeger, and S. Rosseau, *Clin Exp Immunol* 116(2), 340 (1999).
71. L. Bretagne, I.-D. Diatta, M. Faouzi, A. Nobile, M. Bongiovanni, L. P. Nicod, and R. Lazor, *Respiration* 91, 486 (2016).
72. Y. Kotetsu, T. Yanagihara, K. Suzuki, H. Ando, D. Eto, K. Hata, M. Arimura-Omori, Y. Yamamoto, E. Harada, and N. Hamada, *Biomedicines* 9(9), 1231 (2021).
73. C. N. Magee, O. Boenisch, and N. Najafian, *Am J Transplant* 12(10), 2588 (2012).
74. M. D'Alessandro, L. Bergantini, F. Mezzasalma, E. Conticini, D. Cavallaro, S. Gangi, S. Cattelan, E. Bargagli, and P. Cameli, *Mol Diagn Ther* 26(4), 437–449 (2022).
75. A. Moretta, E. Ciccone, G. Tambussi, C. Bottino, O. Viale, D. Pende, A. Santoni, and M. C. Mingari, *Int J Cancer Suppl* 4, 48 (1989).
76. L. Bergantini, M. d'Alessandro, P. Cameli, A. Otranto, T. Finco, G. Curatola, P. Sestini, and E. Bargagli, *Clin Immunol* 230, 108827 (2021).
77. J. H. Kim, H. Y. Kim, S. Kim, J.-H. Chung, W. S. Park, and D. H. Chung, *Am J Pathol* 167(5), 1231 (2005).

4

BAL as a diagnostic tool

SAMANTHA KING, EMILY DECURTIS, TERRI LEBO, JENA TISDALE,
JANE BAER, YONGBAO WANG, MONA RIZEQ, AMY FREY, BRYAN BORG,
AND EDWARD D CHAN

PRE-ANALYTICAL PHASE: USEFULNESS, COLLECTING, AND PROCESSING OF BAL FLUID

Usefulness of BAL fluid

Bronchoalveolar lavage (BAL) is a semi-invasive procedure which allows for sampling of the lower respiratory tract to assist in the diagnosis of lung diseases. The first BAL was performed via a rigid bronchoscope in 1927 (1). With the development of the flexible bronchoscope in 1966, BAL has become a common, relatively safe procedure performed mostly under conscious sedation (2). The BAL fluid can be analyzed by various tests to help diagnose, narrow the differential diagnosis, or rule out certain lung disorders. BAL can be diagnostic, e.g., the presence of malignant cells, microbes that are not part of the normal lung flora such as *Mycobacterium tuberculosis*, or diffuse alveolar hemorrhage as evinced by sequentially bloodier return. BAL fluid can also serve as a sufficient surrogate for lung biopsy in the proper situation, e.g., *(i)* high BAL lymphocytosis and typical radiographic findings for hypersensitivity pneumonitis (with known organic antigen exposure) or for sarcoidosis, *(ii)* characteristic cells consistent with pulmonary Langerhans cell histiocytosis, or *(iii)* copious amounts of Periodic acid–Schiff (PAS)-positive material characteristic of pulmonary alveolar proteinosis. BAL can often help narrow the differential diagnosis, i.e., different sets of diagnoses are characterized by the presence of lymphocytic, eosinophilic, or neutrophilic cellular patterns in the BAL fluid.

Collecting BAL fluid

The fiberoptic bronchoscope is introduced either through the nose, mouth, or endotracheal tube and advanced past the oropharynx, through the vocal folds, and into the airways. The tip of the bronchoscope is then "wedged" (gently occluding the lumen) in the lobar or segmental airway of interest. The area targeted for lavage is typically predetermined based on chest imaging. In the absence of a parenchymal abnormality on chest imaging, the middle lobe or lingula are most often targeted for sampling because, in the supine patient, their relative superior position to

DOI: 10.1201/9781003146834-5

the tip of the bronchoscope leads to greater fluid recovery due to facilitation by gravity. Since the instilled fluid contacts any lung tissue distal to the wedged bronchoscope, the collected sample contains material distal to the bronchoscope tip, such as non-adherent cells, microorganisms, mucus, surfactant, and phospholipids.

Procedurally, room temperature isotonic saline is instilled in two to four sequential aliquots of 30–60 ml each, totaling 60–240 ml, although interstitial lung disease guidelines recommend no less than 100 ml and no more than 300 ml of lavage be performed (3). Each aliquot is aspirated gently via the syringe and/or through the suction port of the bronchoscope, attempting to avoid visible airway collapse, and collected in sterile syringes and/or specimen cups. At least 30% of the instilled saline should be recovered for accurate analysis and to ensure the sample is representative of distal airspaces and not of bronchi, the latter of which may not necessarily reflect the pathology of any lung imaging abnormalities.

The working-channel diameter of the bronchoscope also determines BAL capacity, and therefore affects how much fluid contacts the lungs ("bronchoscope dead space"). When using a bronchoscope with a larger working-channel lumen, a greater proportion of the collected BAL fluid is airway naïve, having never left the bronchoscope, although this is also modified by the chosen aliquot size. The working-channel diameter can range from 1.7 mm (pediatric scope) to 3.0 mm (therapeutic scope). Despite the similar total length of the bronchoscope and working-channel (~600 mm), a cylindrical 2.0 mm working-channel may have a volume of 1.88 ml whereas a cylindrical 3.0 mm working-channel volume may be 4.24 ml. With two to five aliquots administered, the airway-naïve portion of the BAL fluid may range from 3.8 ml up to 21.2 ml; this estimation becomes more inaccurate with the use of a clamshell-shaped working-channel which allows for suctioning around tools, but which could allow recovery of even greater proportion of airway-naïve BAL fluid. Intuitively, the impact of this airway-naïve BAL fluid is higher with smaller volume aliquots and lower percentage of recovery. For example, if 100 ml of sample is instilled in five aliquots through a larger working-channel,

more than 20% of return could in fact be airway naïve; this has been shown to have significant impact on the yield and accuracy of many tests, including most profoundly, cell count/differential and cytology, but less so for microbial cultures or other pathogen diagnostics (4). Conversely, two aliquots totaling 100 ml using the same working-channel volumes may only contain ~4–9% of airway-naïve fluid. The bronchoscopist should be aware of the presence of airway-naïve BAL fluid and the effect it may have on diagnostic yield, with smaller aliquots potentially having the most drastic effects on accuracy.

Processing of BAL fluid in the pre-analytical phase

Following collection in a sterile container(s), BAL fluid should be transported as soon as possible from the bedside or bronchoscopy suite to the clinical laboratory. Generally, the goal transport time should be ≤3–4 hours for BAL cellular analysis (cell differential and flow cytometry), ≤2 hours for microbiology, and ≤24 hours for molecular diagnostics. If greater delay is anticipated, consider transporting on ice. Delay in transportation greater than 2 hours may result in decreased recovery of fastidious pathogens and overgrowth of normal flora (5). Upon receipt of the BAL fluid in the laboratory, it should be treated as infectious and processed using appropriate personal protection equipment in an appropriate biological safety level cabinet. Record the BAL fluid volume (ml). Volume instilled and recovered will be needed for calculation of cell counts. Note the color (e.g., colorless, white, red, brown, pink) and clarity (e.g., clear, slightly cloudy, grossly cloudy, opaque) of the BAL fluid. The BAL sample must be adequately labeled with two patient identifiers, e.g., name and medical record number. If there are multiple sources, e.g., left upper lobe or right lower lobe, etc., the origin should be noted. Transfer BAL fluid into a sterile polypropylene tube using a sterile transfer pipette. Sample volume varies depending on the test to be performed: cell count (2 ml), bacterial/fungal culture (1 ml), acid-fast bacteria culture (1 ml), cytology (1 ml for slide), lymphocyte phenotyping by flow cytometry (15 ml minimum with the exact volume required dependent on lymphocyte count), and beryllium lymphocyte proliferation assay (50 ml preferred).

BAL fluid can be evaluated with a variety of analytical tests including cell counts and differential, cytopathologic analysis, and cultures as well as specific molecular and immunologic diagnostic tests.

BAL CELLULAR ANALYSIS

BAL cell count and differential

CLINICAL VALUE OF BAL CELL COUNT AND DIFFERENTIAL

In healthy non-smokers, macrophages make up about 85–90% of all leukocytes in BAL fluid; lymphocytes 10–15%, neutrophils 3%, and eosinophils and basophils <1% each. Smokers have increased absolute cell counts compared to non-smokers and their differentials tend to have macrophages >90% (often tobacco-product pigmented), lower lymphocyte counts (often <5%), and similar percentages of other leukocyte types (6). BAL cell differentials greater than 15% lymphocytes, 3% neutrophils, 1% eosinophils, or 0.5% mast cells are abnormal and have diagnostic implications. These thresholds lead to the BAL designation as "lymphocytic" or "neutrophilic" cellular pattern. While the BAL cellular pattern is sometimes referred to as a "predominance" of that cell type (e.g., "lymphocyte predominant"), the term "cellular pattern" is preferred since the increased percentage of a particular cell type may be <50%; e.g., a sample with 20% lymphocytes and 55% macrophages is more accurately labeled as lymphocytic cellular pattern.

Although the cell differential findings on BAL often lack specificity, they may assist clinicians in supporting a particular diagnosis or excluding others. For example, the presence of alveolar hemorrhage, high percentage of eosinophils, or lymphocytic cellular pattern can narrow the differential diagnosis. Furthermore, the BAL cell count differential may evolve over time, changing with the stage of the disease process such as in hypersensitivity pneumonitis (i.e., lymphocytosis with moderate neutrophilia with neutrophils declining with time after antigen exposure) (7)

and acute respiratory distress syndrome at varying clinical stages (i.e., early ARDS reveals mostly neutrophils but in the later resolution phases, there are fewer neutrophils and a higher restored number of macrophages) (8, 9). However, the differential cell count may be normal in quiescent chronic obstructive pulmonary disease and asthma or even some cases of drug-induced pneumonitis (10, 11). In some circumstances, no characteristic cell count and differential patterns are discernable, either because of variability of cell counts seen in the disease process, more than one process occurring in the lungs, poor BAL yield (volume or site that may not be representative of process), or limited data on BAL cell counts reported in the literature (12). Hence, transbronchial biopsy and especially surgical lung biopsy retain a prominent role in the formal diagnosis of several lung diseases where BAL findings are non-diagnostic (13, 3).

Neutrophilic BAL

In general, diseases associated with a neutrophilic pattern on the BAL fluid include acute interstitial pneumonia, acute respiratory distress syndrome (initial/exudative phase), bacterial pneumonia, cystic fibrosis, granulomatous polyangiitis, and some drug-induced lung disorders (e.g., bleomycin, erlotinib, trastuzumab, and valproic acid) (12).

Lymphocytic BAL

Lung disorders associated with lymphocytic pattern on the BAL fluid include berylliosis, cryoglobulinemia, granulomatous lymphocytic interstitial lung disease, HIV-associated pneumonitis, hypersensitivity pneumonitis, lymphocytic interstitial pneumonia, non-specific interstitial pneumonia, sarcoidosis, tuberculosis, and numerous drug-induced lung disorders; e.g., checkpoint inhibitors such as anti-PD-1 antibody (pembrolizumab, nivolumab, etc.) and anti-PD-L1 antibody (durvalumab, etc.) > anti-CTLA-4 antibody (ipilimumab, tremelimumab), dasatinib, etanercept, etoposide, gold, radiation-induced pneumonitis, everolimus, and sirolimus (12). A lymphocytic BAL pattern with a compatible clinical history and imaging are adequate evidence to support a diagnosis of pulmonary sarcoidosis or hypersensitivity pneumonitis. In these two processes, CD4:CD8 T cell subtyping by flow cytometry can further support one diagnosis over another, with a ratio of >4 highly specific for sarcoidosis if there is an absence of an increased proportion of other leukocyte types in the BAL sample (3).

Eosinophilic BAL

The differential diagnoses of eosinophilic pattern on the BAL fluid include acute and chronic eosinophilic pneumonia, allergic bronchopulmonary aspergillosis, eosinophilic granulomatosis with polyangiitis, parasitic pneumonias (e.g., paragonimiasis, strongyloides), and some drug-induced lung diseases (e.g., carbamazepine, sulfasalazine, etc.). In a patient with an acute alveolar opacification on chest imaging, the presence of significant BAL eosinophils can indicate acute eosinophilic pneumonia with a fair degree of certainty.

PROTOCOL FOR DETERMINING RED BLOOD CELL AND LEUKOCYTE CONCENTRATION AND LEUKOCYTE DIFFERENTIAL IN BAL FLUID

For cell differential, specimens should be analyzed within 3 hours of receipt as the cells will deteriorate rapidly; otherwise, refrigerate specimen at 2–8°C for up to 24 hours before analyzing. Both red blood cell (RBC) and leukocyte number per ml (concentration, aka "count") and leukocyte differential of the BAL fluid are performed manually (14). The method to determine RBC and leukocyte counts in a neat or diluted BAL sample is shown in Table 4.1. The leukocyte differential is performed visually, based on the morphology of the stained leukocytes on a microscope slide loaded with BAL fluid using a slide centrifugation method (Table 4.2).

Flow cytometry

CLINICAL VALUE OF FLOW CYTOMETRIC ANALYSIS

Flow cytometry can enumerate and identify the phenotype of leukocytes (particularly lymphocytes) in the BAL fluid. Typically, CD3, CD4, CD8, and the CD4:CD8 ratio (T cell markers) and occasionally CD19 (B cell marker) are of diagnostic value with certain other markers depending on the specific situation (15). Flow cytometric analyses of BAL leukocyte phenotype have an important role in the evaluation of several lung diseases, including sarcoidosis, hypersensitivity pneumonitis, and lymphoproliferative disorders (16).

Aiding in distinguishing hypersensitivity pneumonitis from sarcoidosis

CD4/CD8 T cell ratios are informative when considering pulmonary sarcoidosis versus hypersensitivity pneumonitis. These two entities share similar chest imaging distribution of upper lobe predominance and a lymphocytic cellular pattern on BAL. Classically, sarcoidosis is more likely when the CD4/CD8 T cell ratio is >4 in the setting of a lymphocytic pattern BAL (3). Conversely, hypersensitivity pneumonitis is typically characterized by a cytotoxic CD8 alveolitis, and thus often manifests with a low CD4/CD8 T cell ratio. The percentages of CD4 and CD8 T cells determined from a BAL fluid correlate well with immunohistochemical staining of lung tissue biopsy (17). However, in a study of 139 patients meeting diagnostic criteria for hypersensitivity pneumonitis, the mean CD4/CD8 T cell ratio was 3.8, with only 34% meeting the classic inverted ratio (<1) (18).

Furthermore, the CD4/CD8 T cell ratio in sarcoidosis can vary with age (19) and fluctuate with chronicity of disease. Gender may also modify this age effect on CD4/CD8 T cell ratio, as the mean CD4/CD8 T cells were 5.8 for healthy nonsmoking women >43 years of age vs 2.1 in women <40 years of age; this age-related effect was not seen in men (20). Hence, a BAL lymphocytic pattern combined with CD4/CD8 T cell ratio is non-specific, and can be suggestive of, but not necessarily diagnostic of, sarcoidosis or hypersensitivity pneumonitis.

Detection of lymphoid cancer

Typically, BAL fluid is evaluated by purely cytomorphologic means, but when attempting to differentiate reactive inflammatory lymphocyte populations from neoplastic ones, flow cytometry provides more diagnostic information, i.e.,

Table 4.1 Determining the WBC and RBC concentrations ("counts") of the BAL fluid

Make note of the appearance of the BAL fluid (e.g., clear vs cloudy, color, bloody) and the lavage volume instilled and the volume recovered. These will be used to calculate percentage recovery and absolute number of cells collected.

Dilution of the BAL fluid with normal saline is based on the gross appearance:

Clear – no dilution; Hazy – 1:10 dilution; Moderately cloudy or bloody – 1:20 dilution; Very cloudy or grossly bloody – 1:100 or more dilution

Mix the neat or diluted BAL fluid sample well and load both sides of the hemocytometer counting chamber (clean with an alcohol pad and allowed to dry) with approximately 10 µL of the BAL fluid. Overfilling or underfilling may compromise the accuracy of the counts.

Place the loaded hemocytometer in a humidity chamber such as a covered petri dish containing a moistened filter paper. Let it sit for about 5 minutes to allow the cells to settle in a single plane.

Examine under the microscope, first at 10X power for acceptability of loading and cell concentration. If improperly filled, cells are overlapping or not evenly distributed, clean the hemocytometer and start again with a different dilution if necessary.

Move to 40X power and phase microscopy to help distinguish RBC from leukocytes. Enumerate the RBCs and leukocytes by counting the leukocytes in the four corner squares and RBCs in the center square as shown below, noting that the four large corner blue squares are where the WBC is counted, and the small five small red squares are where the RBC is counted. Thus, count the number of leukocytes in each of the four large blue squares and average the number. The leukocyte concentration ($\times 10^6$/ml) = (average number of leukocytes per large blue square $\times$ 10 $\times$ 0.001 $\times$ dilution factor) where 10 is the depth correction factor and 0.001 is the mm^3 correction factor. Similarly, count the number of RBCs in each of the small squares (colored in red) and average the number in each small square. The RBC concentration ($\times 10^6$/ml) = (average number of RBC $\times$ 5 $\times$ 10 $\times$ 0.001 $\times$ dilution factor) where 5 is the correction factor for the red cell area (1/5 of large square).

areas of the grid where WBC are counted

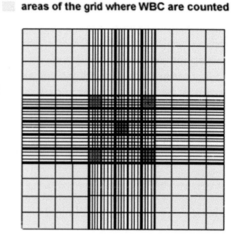

areas of the grid where RBC are counted

Note 1: For cells on the edges, count only the ones on the top or right line of each small square to avoid double counting cells.

Note 2: Multiplying the cell concentration by the volume recovered gives the total number of cells in the sample.

flow cytometry has been demonstrated to be more sensitive than cell morphology in detection of hematolymphoid neoplasms such as leukemia or lymphoma, especially in a paucicellular sample such as a fine needle aspirate (21). In a study of 44 patients with known lymphoproliferative disorders, adding flow cytometry to cytomorphologic analysis of BAL fluid improved the detection rate (22). All 44 BAL samples yielded a diagnosis, but in nine of the cases, there was discordance where the diagnosis was detected by one method but not the other. Flow cytometry detected a lymphoproliferative disorder in eight of these nine, improving the sensitivity of detection from BAL (22). Thus, if there is clinical suspicion for lymphoproliferative disorder, BAL fluid may be submitted for flow cytometry to determine the immunophenotype of the lymphocytes, but the suspicion of

Table 4.2 Determining the WBC differential with stained cytospin slides

Place labeled slide and funnel in the clamp and into the cytofuge.

Dilution of the BAL fluid depends on the WBC concentration obtained. The reason for dilution is to achieve a monolayer of cells so that they are distinguishable from each other.

- If WBC count is ≤20 × 10^6/ml, load 100 μL of the neat BAL to the cytofunnel chamber.
- If WBC count is 20–30 × 10^6/ml, dilute 1:2 with normal saline and load 100 μL of the diluted BAL fluid to the cytofunnel chamber.
- If WBC count is >30 × 10^6/ml, dilute 1:4 with normal saline and load 100 μL of the diluted BAL fluid to the cytofunnel chamber.
- Adding a drop of 22% albumin can help stabilize cells so they don't distort (optional).

Centrifuge slides according to manufacturer's protocol (e.g., 1,000 rpm for 3 minutes).

Remove slide and allow to dry. Stain slide with Wrights or Wrights–Giemsa as desired according to manufacturer's protocol. View the slide via direct microscopy at 100X with oil.

Perform a differential by counting 100 leukocytes (if possible – or count all cells present and adjust accordingly) to obtain percentage of each type of leukocyte (macrophage, lymphocyte, neutrophil, eosinophil).

Macrophages: after Papanicolaou staining, their nuclei appear round to oval, and nuclear size can increase in the setting of acute infection. Their cytoplasm stains gray-green and may contain particles of engulfed material such as hemosiderin, lipid droplets, or tobacco-related inclusions.

Lymphocytes: ~10 μM in diameter with a high nucleus-to-cytoplasm ratio.

Eosinophils: spherical cells with pale blue bi-lobed nuclei and coarse intracellular granules that stain orange/pink on Wrights-Giemsa).

Basophils: Basophils have large dark purple granules mostly obscuring a large nucleus.

Multiply the percentage of each cell type by the WBC count to obtain the absolute numbers of each cell type.

If more slides are needed for cytology – see that section for instructions.

---

such a diagnosis and specific markers to test for should be discussed with a pathologist.

Usefulness of flow cytometry on BAL fluid in other examples of specific lung disorders

When considering a diagnosis of pulmonary Langerhans cell histiocytosis, flow cytometric detection of a CD1(+) monocyte-derived dendritic cell population >5% is often considered diagnostic (23). However, in an analysis of patients with this disease, only 5/15 had >5% of cells positive by flow cytometry, 3/15 had 1–5%, and 7/15 had CD1(+) populations <1% (24). This relation is also modified by current smoking status, where active smoking was somewhat more likely to yield a diagnosis by BAL flow cytometry (24). In this disease, transbronchial lung biopsy or surgical biopsy will likely have higher yield for diagnosis than BAL (25).

In a BAL cell differential study of a relatively large number of subjects, it was found that the likelihood for usual interstitial pneumonitis doubled from a modest 16% to 33% when lymphocytes were <30% with elevated neutrophils (24).

In asthma, the determination of a T_H2 high versus low pattern of inflammation may have impacts on treatment options and prognosis. T_H2 high inflammation is associated with elevated intracellular interleukin-4 (IL-4), IL-5, and IL-13 which recruit a population of eosinophils, dendritic cells, mast cells, and basophils that may be detected by their cell markers on flow cytometry (26, 27). High levels of these markers may help the clinician to determine the likelihood of a positive response to a given asthma treatment plan, and in the future may allow a more personalized approach to treatment.

PRE-ANALYTICAL COLLECTION, TRANSPORT, AND STORAGE OF BAL SAMPLE FOR FLOW CYTOMETRY

Flow cytometry should be performed on fresh cells within 4 hours of sample collection as cells in BAL fluid can rapidly deteriorate after this timeframe. If timely analysis of the BAL fluid is not possible, centrifuge the specimen at $514 \times g$ at room temperature for 5–7 minutes. Discard the supernatant and replace with RPMI medium supplemented with Pen-Strep, L-glutamine, and AB serum (10%) and store at 2–8°C, until processing can take place (preferably within 24 hours). Specimens >4 hours old should have a viability test performed by diluting the sample with trypan blue (0.4%) at 1:1 ratio; if cell suspension is too concentrated, dilute it in PBS buffer sufficiently so that the cells are not overlapping in the chamber. This dilution is loaded onto the hemocytometer as in the section on BAL cell count and differential. Load both sides of the hemocytometer with the dilution and after the cells have settled (~3 minutes), count 100 cells on each side of the chamber, and obtain an average percentage of viable cells. While it is preferred that specimens have at least an 80% viability, useful information may still be gathered on suboptimal specimens. Staining should still be performed on suboptimal BAL specimens (since repeating a bronchoscopy to obtain the BAL fluid is not practical) but the decreased viability should be noted in the report.

CALIBRATION AND CONTROLS FOR FLOW CYTOMETRY

There are several flow cytometers available from various manufacturers capable of detecting four to eight different fluorochromes or more (= number of fluorochrome-tagged antibodies). Those that are Food and Drug Administration (FDA) approved for clinical purposes have instructions for optimal performance assessment and standardization. The cytometer must be appropriately calibrated, typically with fluorochromes attached to latex beads that may be vendor specific. Furthermore, appropriate control material(s) should be run at specified intervals. For clinical laboratories, there are stringent regulatory requirements that must be met regarding instrumentation, reagents, control materials, protocols, and validation of assays. It is advisable to be familiar with these before proceeding.

There are several types of controls used in flow cytometry. Method controls are samples of known antigenicity that are processed in conjunction with the clinical (BAL) sample to ensure all antibodies and processing steps have been added/completed appropriately. Several companies sell preserved cell solutions of a known type and number that can be utilized; however, preservatives do affect fluorescence so this must be taken into consideration. These have the advantage of a longer shelf life – generally about 30 days and the ability to monitor their performance over time to look for shifts or trends that could indicate instrument problems. Fresh whole blood or frozen peripheral blood mononuclear cell preparations may also be used as method controls. Internal controls consist of populations known to be negative for an antigen, e.g., CD19, a marker for B cells is not present on T cells, and thus T cells can serve as a negative control for the B cell marker (28). Another internal control is calculating the total percentage of lymphocytes (aka "lymphosum"), i.e., the percentages of T cells + B cells + NK cells should equal approximately 100% of lymphocytes.

PROCESSING OF BAL SAMPLE FOR FLOW CYTOMETRY

Some of the basic reagents, supplies, and equipment for using the flow cytometer are listed in Table 4.3. BAL fluid tends to be very messy, containing mucus, clumps of cells, and bacteria. The flow cell on a flow cytometer is very small, with cells passing through single file; therefore, it can easily become clogged with debris. Thus, BAL fluids should be filtered prior to processing with a 70 μm cell strainer to remove these clogging items while retaining most leukocytes. Additionally, an added protein source such as AB serum will help to keep the cells intact.

The amount of BAL fluid needed depends on the leukocyte concentration but in general about 200 μL of 1×10^6 cells/ml will be needed. Centrifuge sufficient volume of BAL fluid to achieve this concentration at 514 x g for 5–7

Table 4.3 Reagents, supplies, and equipment for flow cytometry

Fluorochrome-labeled antibody cocktails (premixed) for CD3/CD4/CD8 T cells and CD19 B cells such as those available from BD Biosciences or Beckman Coulter.

Lysing solution available from commercial vendors such as BD or Beckman Coulter.

Trypan blue (0.4%) for viability testing.

RPMI supplemented with 10% Human AB serum, penicillin-Streptomycin /L-glutamine (suitable for cell culture media preparation) used for transport/storage of aged specimens.

Human AB serum or suitable protein source.

Cell strainer (70 μm) for filtering mucus from BAL fluid.

Centrifuge with swing bucket rotor and carriers to fit 12 × 75mm tubes.

Pipettes and tips capable of dispensing 2–1,000 μL.

Hemocytometer and coverslips (for viability testing).

Vortexer.

12 × 75 mm polystyrene tubes (Falcon or equivalent).

50 ml polypropylene tubes (Falcon or equivalent).

Flow cytometer capable of 4–6 color fluorescence detection and appropriate software. BD Biosciences and Beckman Coulter have FDA-approved instruments that may be used for this purpose.

minutes. Discard the supernatant and reconstitute the pellet with 200 μL of AB serum.

Premixed antibody cocktails for CD45, CD3, CD4, CD8, CD19, and CD16/56 are available from several manufacturers. Often these have specific processing instructions. Follow the manufacturer's staining protocol for the volume of antibiotic cocktail and cell suspension to aliquot (e.g., 20 μL of antibody cocktail to 50 μL cell suspension) into 12 × 75 mm polystyrene tubes (glass and polypropylene tubes are not acceptable as the tubes will be pressurized in the instrument). Vortex the preparations and incubate at room temperature in the dark for an appropriate amount of time (e.g., 15 minutes), add an appropriate amount of lysing solution (e.g., 450 μL but vendor dependent), vortex again, and incubate at room temperature in the dark (e.g., 15 minutes). If the lysing solution also contains a fixative (vendor dependent), then the sample is now ready to be acquired on the calibrated flow cytometer, along with control(s); otherwise, store at 2–8°C (for up to about three days) until ready to read. Washing steps with PBS for the preparation during the staining process is typically not required for FDA-approved clinical testing systems; however, vendor instructions should be followed as appropriate instrument settings (PMT voltages

and compensation) will differ depending on the type of preparation.

ACQUISITION AND ANALYSIS OF THE FLOW CYTOMETER

Clinical instruments typically have software specifically designed to acquire and analyze whole blood and/or other body fluids for T, B, and NK cells; while this streamlines the process, non-clinical software may also be used. In the latter case, it is advisable to set up acquisition and analysis templates for consistent results. The following dot-plot flow cytometric diagram of an actual BAL sample demonstrates lymphocyte analysis using one manufacturer's template which was designed for whole blood but was adapted and validated for BAL fluid. The initial dot-plot sorts the cells based on the pan leukocyte marker (CD45) on the x-axis and side scatter (function of intracellular complexity of the cells) on the y-axis (Figure 4.1A). Lymphocytes are "gated" or isolated using CD45(+) cells that also possess low side scatter as lymphocytes are less complex internally than monocytes or granulocytes; thus, the lymphocyte population in the BAL fluid is identified by the cells outlined at the bottom of the y-axis (Figure 4.1A). Lymphocytes are split into CD3(+) T cells and CD3(–) B

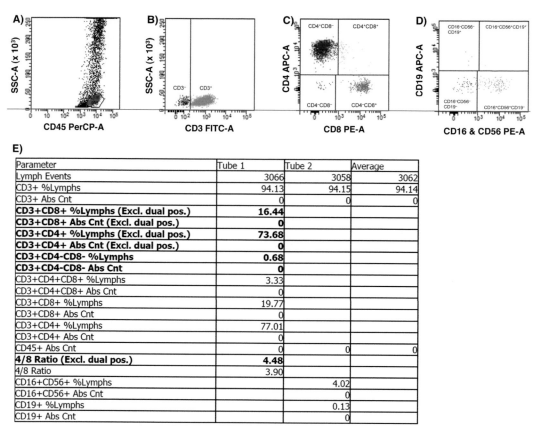

Figure 4.1 Flow cytometric analysis of a BAL fluid sample. (A) Dot-plot of cells sorted by side scatter (SSC-A) on the y-axis and the pan leukocyte marker CD45 on the x-axis. Lymphocytes are identified by high levels of CD45(+) cells with low side scatter (outlined cells on the dot-plot). (B) Dot-plot of cells sorted by side scatter (SSC-A) on the y-axis and the T cell marker CD3 on the x-axis. CD3(+) T lymphocytes are identified as high CD3(+) and low side scatter. (C) The CD3(+) T cells are sorted as CD4(+) or CD8(+) T cells. Tube 1 of BAL cell suspension is stained with fluoro-chrome-labeled anti-CD45 antibody, anti-CD3(+) antibody, anti-CD4(+) antibody, and anti-CD8(+) antibody. Plots A, B, and C reflect what is in Tube 1. (D) Dot-plot of BAL cells sorted by B cell marker (CD19) and NK cell markers (CD16 and CD56). Tube 2 of BAL cell suspension is stained with fluorochrome-labeled anti-CD45 antibody, anti-CD3(+) antibody, anti-CD19 antibody, anti-CD16(+) antibody, and anti-CD56(+) antibody. Plots A, B, and D reflect what is in Tube 2. (E) Table denotes the percentage of the aforementioned lymphocyte subsets. The bold results in E (Table) are for New York state reporting only.

and NK cells (Figure 4.1B). CD3(+) T cells are further divided into CD4 and CD8 T cell subsets (Figure 4.1C) whereas CD3(−) B and NK cells are differentiated with CD19 and CD16/56, respectively (Figure 4.1D). These results are percentages of lymphocyte subsets. Absolute numbers of cell subsets may be derived by multiplying the subset percentage by the absolute lymphocyte count obtained in the cell count and differential.

The ratio of CD4:CD8 T cells is also a useful parameter. Typical BAL samples, unless they are contaminated with peripheral blood, should have few, if any, B or NK cells present. Large numbers of B cells in the absence of peripheral blood contamination could indicate a lymphoproliferative disorder. In such cases, a pathologist should be consulted regarding further investigation with additional markers. If a viability test was

E)

Parameter	Tube 1	Tube 2	Average
Lymph Events	3066	3058	3062
CD3+ %Lymphs	94.13	94.15	94.14
CD3+ Abs Cnt	0	0	0
CD3+CD8+ %Lymphs (Excl. dual pos.)	**16.44**		
CD3+CD8+ Abs Cnt (Excl. dual pos.)	**0**		
CD3+CD4+ %Lymphs (Excl. dual pos.)	**73.68**		
CD3+CD4+ Abs Cnt (Excl. dual pos.)	**0**		
CD3+CD4-CD8- %Lymphs	**0.68**		
CD3+CD4-CD8- Abs Cnt	**0**		
CD3+CD4+CD8+ %Lymphs	3.33		
CD3+CD4+CD8+ Abs Cnt	0		
CD3+CD8+ %Lymphs	19.77		
CD3+CD8+ Abs Cnt	0		
CD3+CD4+ %Lymphs	77.01		
CD3+CD4+ Abs Cnt	0		
CD45+ Abs Cnt	0	0	0
4/8 Ratio (Excl. dual pos.)	**4.48**		
4/8 Ratio	3.90		
CD16+CD56+ %Lymphs		4.02	
CD16+CD56+ Abs Cnt		0	
CD19+ %Lymphs		0.13	
CD19+ Abs Cnt		0	

performed, this percentage should be included in the report.

BAL cytology

SPECIMEN SUBMISSION

Prior to the BAL procedure, clinical determination of which studies are necessary should be made so that the specimen is submitted to the laboratory appropriately fresh and/or in fixative. The studies requested should be clearly communicated, particularly if several studies are needed to ensure appropriate handling in the various laboratory departments (Clinical Laboratory vs Cytology Department). For example, the specimen should be submitted fresh for cell count, flow cytometry and microbiologic studies, and Oil red O staining whereas BAL specimens submitted for cytologic examination only are ideally submitted in a fixative. The fixative used varies depending on the methodology used by the laboratory, e.g., Cytolyte® fixative is used by some labs.

If Oil red O staining is needed in addition to cytologic evaluation, then the BAL must be submitted fresh so that the Oil red O stain can be done prior to adding fixative to the specimen for the cytologic evaluation. If submitted fresh, the BAL specimen should be transported as soon as possible following acquisition to the cytology laboratory where the specimen can be refrigerated for up to 24–48 hours prior to processing.

Processing and staining methods will vary depending on whether these are done manually or using automated instruments. If there is sufficient cellularity, a cell block can be made in addition to the cytospin, allowing for special stains and immunohistochemical stains to be performed.

USES OF BAL CYTOLOGY

Cytologic examination of the BAL is primarily for detection of malignant cells, acellular entities, or infectious organisms (e.g., *Pneumocystis jirovecii* and sulfur granules (29)) (Table 4.4) and rarely for Oil red O staining (e.g., for amiodarone compliance).

Malignancy detection

The sensitivity for detection of malignancy by BAL varies depending on the site and extent of

Table 4.4 Cells, acellular entities, and organisms that may be seen on cytologic examination

Cells
Squamous and glandular cells (benign and
  malignant)
Acute and chronic inflammatory cells
Alveolar macrophages
Acellular entities
Hemosiderin (in macrophages)
Curschmann's spirals
Charcot-Leyden crystals
Anthracotic pigment
Lipid droplets (in macrophages)
Contaminants (e.g., talc)
Ferruginous bodies
Exudate characteristic of pulmonary alveolar
  proteinosis
Organisms
Pneumocystis jirovecii
Sulfur granules containing actinomyces and/or
  other types of bacteria

the tumor and whether the tumor is diffuse or multifocal (higher sensitivity) (30) or peripheral and not seen on bronchoscopy (lower sensitivity) (31). The sensitivity and specificity of a single BAL sample in one report was 48% compared to 65% on bronchial brushing and 89% on fine needle aspiration (32).

It is essential that clinical and radiologic information accompanies the specimen to assist with the diagnosis since pitfalls in interpretation include reactive cellular responses with marked atypia that may simulate malignancy, e.g., radiation/chemotherapy-associated changes, pulmonary infarcts, infections, diffuse alveolar damage, and bone marrow transplantation (33, 34).

Cellular stains

Special stains and immunohistochemical stains can be performed on cell blocks if there is sufficient cellularity. Such staining may enhance more specific differentiation of the tumor type if this is not evident in the cytomorphologic features alone. Immunohistochemical stains can be helpful in determining the primary site of the tumor; however, these are infrequently specific since they may show reactivity in a number of tumor types, albeit in different percentages, and hence clinical and radiologic correlations are always necessary.

The Papanicolaou (Pap) stain is the most widely used stain for the cytologic study of cells in BAL fluid (Figure 4.2A/B) although the standard H&E stain may provide an initial clue for the presence of cancer cells (Figure 4.2C). It stains nuclear chromatin with differential cytoplasmic staining allowing for the evaluation of nuclear features (hyperchromasia, nuclear membrane irregularity in malignant cells vs uniform fine chromatin pattern with smooth regular nuclear membranes for non-malignant cells) and cytoplasmic quality (dense eosinophilic cytoplasm suggesting squamous differentiation, vacuolated pale cytoplasm and intracytoplasmic lumina suggesting glandular differentiation). Pap staining is often done by automation, but a manual back-up method is shown in Table 4.5.

Periodic acid–Schiff (PAS), PAS diastase (PAS-D), and/or mucicarmine stains are used to detect the presence of mucin in an adenocarcinoma. Some examples of specific malignancies and cell markers used to identify them include: *(i)* lymphoma (leukocyte common antigen positive); *(ii)* carcinoma (cytokeratin positive); *(iii)* non-small cell lung carcinoma (adenocarcinomas are TTF-1 (Figure 4.2D) and Napsin A positive and squamous cell carcinomas are p40 positive); *(iv)* small cell carcinoma (CD56 positive). Differentiating primary from metastatic carcinoma in the BAL will depend on what other primaries are clinical

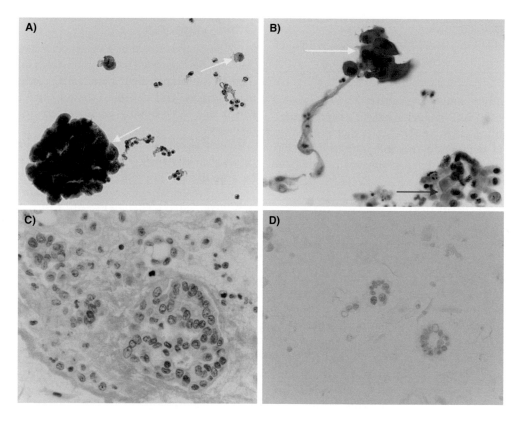

Figure 4.2 Detection of malignant cells in the BAL fluid. (A) Pap stain (40X). Top right arrow: benign bronchial epithelial cell with cilia (stained light red). Lower left arrow: Adenocarcinoma (malignant cells with nuclear enlargement and overlapping, irregular chromatin pattern and multiple nucleoli). (B) Pap stain (60X). Cohesive cluster of malignant squamous cells with dense eosinophilic cytoplasm. (C) H&E stain of a BAL cell block (60X). The acinar structure is consistent with an adenocarcinoma. (D) Thyroid transcription factor-1 (TTF-1) immunostain (40X). The positive nuclear stain in the adenocarcinoma supports a lung primary.

Table 4.5 Papanicolaou staining protocol (manual)

Reagent	Number of dips/ Time in reagent
95% reagent alcohol	10 dips
Tap or DI water	10 dips
Hematoxylin	4 minutes
Tap or DI water	10 dips
Bluing solution	10 dips
Tap or DI water	10 dips
95% reagent alcohol	20 dips
Orange G-6	1 minute
95% reagent alcohol	10 dips
95% reagent alcohol	10 dips
EA50	2 minutes
95% reagent alcohol	20 dips
100% reagent alcohol	20 dips
Citrus clearing solvent	20 dips
Citrus clearing solvent	3 minutes, hold until mounting

possibilities: lung (cytokeratin 7 [CK7]), colon (CK20, CDX2), bladder (GATA3), thyroid (thyroglobulin), prostate (NKX3.1), melanoma (Sox 10), and neuroendocrine differentiation (CD56, chromogranin, and synaptophysin positivity to varying degrees).

Infection detection

BAL is also useful in the identification of infections, particularly in immunosuppressed individuals and in combination with microbiologic studies. A portion of the specimen is submitted fresh for microbiologic studies with a portion in fixative for cytologic examination.

Gram stain, Grocott–Gomori's methenamine silver (GMS) stain, and acid-fast stain can identify the presence of infectious organisms (bacterial, fungal, or mycobacterial, respectively) if the sample is representative and contains sufficient organisms. However, microbiologic studies are also essential.

Infections on routine Pap-stained slides from the BAL may show non-specific features such as acute inflammation and reparative bronchial epithelial cell changes. In addition, some infections exhibit characteristic and diagnostic viral cytopathic effects, e.g., cytomegalovirus (nuclear enlargement with intranuclear inclusions); herpes simplex virus (multinucleation with nuclear molding and margination). Immunohistochemical stains on cell block material can confirm these diagnoses if the cytomorphologic features are indeterminate.

Pneumocystis jirovecii appear as blue-green granular casts within which there are refractile disc-shaped or clear spaces; the presence of organisms can be confirmed on GMS stains which will highlight the crescent-shaped or round organisms. Since there may be very few organisms, particularly if the patient has already been treated, identification may be best done using direct fluorescence antibody which can detect *P. jirovecii* infection as this organism does not grow on culture media.

Other diagnoses

Sarcoidosis and fungal and mycobacterial infections are characterized by granulomatous inflammation (multinucleated giant cells, epithelioid macrophages, and chronic inflammatory cells), which may occasionally be identified on BAL cytology.

Stains may also be used for noninfectious processes such as alveolar proteinosis, characterized by granular eosinophilic (PAS positive diastase resistant) material, multi-nucleated foreign body type giant cells, positive Oil red O (if material is submitted fresh for staining), and negative mucicarmine.

MICROBIOLOGIC ANALYSIS

Microbiologic value of the BAL fluid

Infections in the lower respiratory tract are the ninth leading cause of mortality in the United States (35). BAL is often performed to obtain respiratory samples in suspected infections for microbiologic culture and analysis when patients are unable to expectorate sputum, even after an attempt at sputum induction, or to rule out active infection when an autoimmune or other inflammatory lung disease is of concern as these diseases often require immunosuppressive medications. Depending on the institution and provider, BAL is used relatively frequently to diagnose ventilator-associated pneumonia (VAP), particularly in immunocompromised patients (36, 37). Quantitative bacterial culture from BAL has a sensitivity of 82–91% when the $\geq 10^4$ colony-forming units (CFU)/ml cutoff for primary pathogen identification is used (38). Culture is also essential to test for antibiotic resistance. The accuracy of BAL in diagnosing certain infections may be compromised due to prior administration of antibiotics (39), poor culture yield on certain fastidious organisms, and/or dilution of the sample.

The potential antimicrobial activity of topical lidocaine has been reviewed (40). While local anesthetics may possess inherent antimicrobial activity, it is important to distinguish the clinical setting or the experimental conditions under which the studies were conducted since, for example, the effects of lidocaine on a wound culture may be quite different from that of a BAL culture since there would be a significant dilution effect of the anesthetic concentration in the latter instance by the lavaged fluid. Another important caveat is distinguishing the effects of lidocaine in purely *in vitro* studies vs studies that examine the effects of lidocaine given *in vivo*. In a purely *in vitro* study, a final 1% lidocaine inhibited the growth of *Staphylococcus aureus*, *Escherichia coli*, and *Pseudomonas aeruginosa*, corroborating its intrinsic antimicrobial effects (41) whereas in another *in vitro* study, lidocaine (and other local anesthetics) had no effect on the growth of *S. aureus*, *Staphylococcus epidermidis*, or *Bacillus subtilis* (42). These differences may be related to differences in the different *in vitro* techniques, e.g., lidocaine added directly to liquid culture wherein the lidocaine concentration is certain (41) vs lidocaine-impregnated discs where the actual lidocaine concentration diffusing from the discs into the agar is essentially unknown (42). In an *ex vivo* study in which bacterial isolates were added to normal saline or BAL fluid obtained from a healthy individual (in which 15–20 ml of 2% lidocaine was used in the bronchoscopic procedure), there was no difference in the growth of spiked *Haemophilus influenzae*, *P. aeruginosa*, or *Candida albicans* but there was significant inhibition of two of four *Streptococcus pneumoniae* isolates by the BAL fluid (containing lidocaine administered *in vivo*) compared

to normal saline (43). One caveat to this study is that it is plausible that the BAL fluid contained other substances (such as endogenous antimicrobial peptides) that could have also inhibited the *S. pneumoniae* growth. For example, in this study the BAL fluid was previously frozen, then thawed (not a normal practice in processing of BAL fluid for microbial detection) (43); this process may have released leukocyte components which were inhibitory to *S. pneumoniae*. However, a separate study in which bronchial fluid (not lavage) from 130 patients was obtained before and after administration of 2% lidocaine showed no difference in culture results before and after *in vivo* lidocaine administration in the 60 patients with positive cultures (44). In summary, the lidocaine administered *in vivo* during a bronchoscopy has the potential to inhibit microbial growth but the degree and significance it does so in individual cases are uncertain due to many uncontrollable variables.

Newer diagnostic techniques including polymerase chain reaction (PCR) and other molecular assays enhance the role of BAL in identifying specific microbial infections. Among immunocompromised patients who are vulnerable to a wider range of pathogens and may not exhibit classic symptoms or radiographic findings, early BAL is particularly useful, especially when combined with cytology staining, as in the case of *P. jirovecii* pneumonia where the organism does not grow on culture. Additionally, more recent diagnostic techniques such as matrix-assisted laser desorption/ionization time-of-flight mass spectrometry (MALDI-TOF) and PCR coupled to electrospray ionization mass spectrometry (PCR/ESI-MS) both show potential to provide rapid microbiologic results of BAL fluid that will enable clinicians to target particular organisms far sooner than conventionally possible (45, 46). More recently, whole-genome sequencing, including real-time metagenomic sequencing (often termed Shotgun Metagenomic Sequencing (SMS)) of BAL fluid has been used to diagnose and manage viral, bacterial, and fungal pneumonias in critically ill patients with and without immunosuppression (47, 48). In addition, SMS of BAL fluid has been used to characterize the metagenomics and microbiome of the respiratory tract of lung transplant recipients (49) and patients with chronic lung diseases (50). As whole-genome sequencing becomes more readily available in clinical laboratories, its role in the analysis of BAL fluid will likely increase.

Basic staining techniques

GRAM STAIN TECHNIQUE

BAL fluid (5–6 drops) is placed onto a glass slide. The slide is placed into a cytospin specimen chamber and centrifuged for 5 minutes at 1,500 rpm to concentrate the fluid. Alternatively, 1–2 drops of BAL can be directly applied to a slide, air dried, and the cells fixed to the slide by heating (42°C for 10 seconds) or applying methanol (which is considered to produce a cleaner background) (51). With methanol fixation, a few drops of methanol are added to the slide and incubated for 1 minute; alternatively, the slide can be dipped into methanol for a few seconds, then allowed to air dry. The most common method used for Gram staining in the clinical setting is Hucker's method (Table 4.6) (52).

Gram-positive organisms have a thick peptidoglycan layer with a large amount of teichoic acid, leaving these organisms unaffected by the decolorizing step. As a result, these organisms will retain the primary crystal violet stain and appear blue/purple. Gram-negative organisms have a thin peptidoglycan layer attached to an asymmetric lipopolysaccharide-phospholipid bilayer outer membrane interrupted with proteins. Thus, alcohol in the decolorizer will damage the outer membrane in Gram-negative organisms, the

Table 4.6 Gram staining procedure

Flood the slide with primary stain, crystal violet solution for 30 seconds.

Rinse the slide with tap water.

Flood the slide with iodine for 30 seconds and then rinse with tap water.

Add alcohol-acetone decolorizer to wash the slide until the fluid runs clear, typically 1–5 seconds. Rinse with tap water.

Flood the slide with counterstain, safranin, for 15–30 seconds. Rinse with tap water.

Once air dried, examine by microscopy.

primary stain will leak out and be replaced by the secondary safranin stain, and the organisms will appear pink/red. To detect bacteria following Gram staining, the slide is observed on low power (10X objective with 10X eye piece) with examination of 20 to 40 fields recommended. The average number of leukocytes observed is semi-quantified. Next, 20 to 40 fields using high power (100X objective with 10X eye piece) are observed. Organisms are typically reported based on: (i) Gram stain characteristics ("positive," "negative," or "variable" where the last term is used when the organisms cannot be grouped as either positive or negative); (ii) morphologic descriptors of "rods" (elongated forms) or "cocci" (rounded forms); (iii) if present, the formation of pairs, chains, or clusters; and (iv) semi-quantitative assessment of the number of organisms using terms such as "few," "moderate," or "many."

ACID-FAST STAIN TECHNIQUE

Although the mycobacterial cell wall contains abundant mycolic acid, the cell wall also contains peptidoglycan, a carbohydrate found in Gram-positive bacteria. While mycobacteria do stain Gram-positive, their peptidoglycan layer is less than other bacteria of this designation and thus Gram-positive staining is weaker with mycobacteria than typical Gram-positive organisms such as *S. aureus* (53, 54). The most common stains used to detect mycobacteria are carbol fuchsin stains such as Kinyoun (no heat-fixing) or Ziehl–Neelsen (heat-fixing required), or fluorochrome stains such as auramine O or auramine-rhodamine (Table 4.7).

Smears are made by placing one drop of the sediment from the decontaminated and concentrated BAL onto a glass slide; the decontamination and concentration procedures are described below. The slide is heat-fixed for 2 hours at 70–80°C; the procedure is performed in a biosafety cabinet to protect the operator from potentially infectious organisms. Thereafter, the specimen is stained with a carbol fuchsin stain, rinsed, and decolorized with 1% sulfuric acid. Those organisms that resist this decolorization process, which include most *Mycobacteria* species, are thus termed "acid-fast." After an additional rinse, the counterstain, methylene blue, is applied.

Table 4.7 Acid-fast staining procedure

Heat-fix the slide for 2 hours at 80°C.	
Carbol fuchsin stain	**Fluorochrome stain**
Flood the slide with primary stain, heat until steaming, and allow stain to sit for 5 minutes	Flood the slide with fluorochrome stain for 15 minutes
Rinse with water	Rinse with water
Flood the slide with 3% acid alcohol for 2 minutes	Flood the slide with 0.5% acid alcohol for 2 minutes
Rinse with water	Rinse with water
Flood the slide with counterstain (methylene blue or brilliant green) for 1 minute	Flood the slide with counterstain (potassium permanganate or acridine orange) for 2 minutes
Once air died, examine with light microscope at 1,000X oil immersion. In a positive stain, the organisms will appear as red rods against a blue or green background, whereas negative will be no red stain present	Once air dried, examine with fluorescent microscope at 450X total magnification. In a positive stain the organisms will appear as yellow or orange rods against a dark background. The amount of AFB present in a stain is reported semi-quantitatively.

Using morphology is important when identifying acid-fast bacilli (AFB) via stains. Usually AFB appear as slender rods, 0.2–0.6 μm wide and 1–10 μm long (55). *Mycobacterium tuberculosis* is typically serpentine cords that clump in liquid culture (a process termed "cording") due to the compound trehalose 6,6′-dimycolate (TDM), a glycolipid also known as "cord factor." Non-tuberculous mycobacteria tend not to form cords, although there are cited exceptions (56). Results are semi-quantified based on the number of acid-fast positive organisms seen per field. It is worth noting that *Nocardia* species, a filamentous bacterium, possesses a mycolic acid layer, although thinner than that of most *Mycobacterium* species. Hence, *Nocardia* do not withstand the harsh decolorization step and, thus, are, typically, not detectable by the acid-fast technique. Therefore, if clinical suspicion warrants testing for *Nocardia*, a weaker acid (typically 1% sulfuric acid) is needed; the acid-fast staining technique using this weaker acid is referred to as the "partial acid-fast" or "modified acid-fast" method (57).

GROCOTT–GOMORI'S METHENAMINE SILVER (GMS) STAIN TECHNIQUE

Many fungi and some bacteria are highlighted when silver solutions are reduced to precipitate silver ions upon the surface of these organisms (termed the "argentaffin reaction"). The stain imparts a black color to the organisms with a light green background. The biochemical reaction involves the following: the mucopolysaccharide components of the fungal cell wall are oxidized to release aldehyde groups. These aldehyde groups then react with the silver nitrate present in the stain, reducing it to a metallic silver, rendering the organisms visible (Table 4.8) (58–60). Like the aforementioned stains, the GMS may be used on fresh BAL or paraffin-embedded cell blocks. This method of identification, though, is relatively non-specific, in that the silver may also highlight non-microbial structures, including plasma proteins including mucins, glycogen, and granules within and from lysed granulocytic leukocytes. The latter may present a problem in differentiating these particles from coccoid bacteria or yeast.

Basic culture techniques

ROUTINE BACTERIAL CULTURE

BAL fluid culture should be quantified, which may be performed either by serial dilution or by the loop method. Serial dilutions should only be inoculated to non-selective media and can be made with saline or phosphate buffer saline (PBS). For example, 50 μL of BAL are transferred to 5 ml

Table 4.8 Grocott–Gomori's methenamine silver (GMS) staining procedure

Deparaffinize and hydrate with distilled water (for cell blocks)

Add 2% chromic acid, microwave at high power for 45 seconds and allow to stand for 5 minutes

Wash in tap water, rinse in distilled water

Flood slide with 1% sodium metabisulfite for 1 minute at room temperature

Wash in tap water, rinse in three changes of distilled water

Add working methenamine silver solution, microwave on high power for 70 seconds. Tissue should be the color of a brown paper bag.

Agitate the slides in the hot solution

Rinse in two changes of distilled water

Add 0.5% gold chloride for 1 minute or until cell block is gray

Wash in distilled water

Add 5% sodium thiosulfate for 3 minutes

Wash in tap water and rinse in distilled water

Incubate slide with working light green solution for 1 minute.

Rinse in distilled water

Rinse slide in progressive concentrations of ethanol (50%, 70%, 80%, 95%, 100% × 2) to dehydrate tissue

Rinse slide with three changes of xylene to remove alcohol from tissue

Add mounting medium to slide and cover slide with coverslip

of PBS to create a 1:100 dilution. Accordingly, 50 μL of the 1:100 dilution transferred to 5 ml of PBS would create a 1:10,000 dilution. Thereafter, 100 μL of the 1:10,000 may be used to inoculate each medium plate. Each colony from these plates, then, equals 10^5 CFU/ml. A more expedient technique, the loop method, is conducted with 0.01 ml and 0.001 ml calibrated loops to inoculate the BAL. Either method uses blood agar (BAP), chocolate agar (CHOC), and either MacConkey agar (MAC) or eosin methylene blue agar (EMB). Buffered charcoal yeast extract agar (BYCE) and BYCE with PAV (polymyxin B, anisomycin, and vancomycin, used to inhibit growth of other bacteria and yeasts) can be added if *Legionella* is suspected. For quantitative colony determination, a disposable rod is used to spread the fluid evenly across the entire media surface. The remaining specimen is then streaked onto the same agar types for isolation. Plates should be incubated at 35–37°C in 5% CO_2 for a minimum of 48 hours with 72 hours preferred. Cultures are then examined after 18–24 hours of incubation, using a Gram stain of the original specimen as a guide to interpreting the culture. Even if growth is identified at 24 hours, cultures should be incubated for an additional 24–48 hours to detect slow-growing and fastidious organisms. After incubation, colonies of pathogens are counted and multiplied by the dilution factor to determine the number of bacteria per ml of BAL. Pathogens may be identified by biochemical or other methods such as MALDI-TOF. Since the lung is not sterile, the clinical significance of an isolated pathogen depends upon the quantitative recovery (Table 4.9).

FUNGAL CULTURE

Potassium hydroxide (KOH) dissolves proteinaceous tissue and allows the fungi to be seen more clearly and calcofluor binds to the chitinous cell wall of fungi and fluoresces under UV light (15). Slides can be made with KOH alone or in combination with calcofluor. One drop of KOH is added to one drop of BAL on a slide, and a coverslip is placed on top. The slide should sit at room temperature for 5–30 minutes before examination. The specimen is examined at 40X for branching hyphae, pseudohyphae, mycelia, and budding yeast forms. If calcofluor is used, a fluorescent microscope is required; fungi will appear yellow-green or blue-green depending upon the filters used. The presence of mycelial structures and hyphae is important for the diagnosis of aspergillosis and other infections caused by mold, especially important for immunocompromised patients. Galactomannan in the BAL is considered to be more sensitive than plasma galactomannan for the diagnosis of invasive aspergillosis. Although *Candida* spp. are often isolated from respiratory secretions (or BAL) of mechanically ventilated patients, detecting *Candida* spp. in respiratory specimens usually

Table 4.9 Significance of bacteria isolated depends on the quantitative culture

Any amount isolated is usually or definitively significant
- *Streptococcus pyogenes* (group A strep)
- *Streptococcus agalactiae* (group B strep) in pediatric patients
- *Streptococcus pneumoniae*
- *Hemophilus influenza*
- *Bordetella* spp., especially, *B. bronchiseptica*
- *Francisella tularensis*
- *Yersinia pestis*
- *Neisseria gonorrhoeae*
- *Nocardia*
- *Bacillus anthracis*
- *Pseudomonas aeruginosa*
- *Stenotrophomonas maltophilia*
- *Acinetobacter baumanni*
- *Burkholderia* spp.
- *Legionella*

Significant amount (>10⁴ CFU/ml)

Significant amount ($>10^4$ CFU/ml)
- *Moraxella catarrhalis*
- *Neisseria meningitidis*
- *Streptococcus agalactiae* (Group B streptococcus), Group C, and Group G streptococcus in adult patients
- *Staphylococcus aureus*
- Single morphotype of Gram-negative rods
- Fastidious Gram-negative rods (e.g., *Pasteurella*)
- *Corynebacterium pseudodiphtheriticum* in immunocompromised patients

Pure or predominant amount
- β-hemolytic streptococci (besides small colony type streptococcus and Group F streptococcus as they are part of the normal upper respiratory tract flora)

>90% of culture
- Coagulase-negative *Staphylococcus*
- *Enterococcus* spp.
- Yeast

represents colonization of the tracheobronchial tree (61). However, if there is no evidence of other infections, isolated *Candida* spp. should be considered as the culprit organisms, especially in immunocompromised hosts. *Candida* spp.

quantities $\geq 10^4$/ml or *Candida glabrata* abundance may also result in positive galactomannan – whether true positive or false positive (62).

There are many types of media that can be used for fungal cultures. For BAL specimens the primary media are brain heart infusion (BHI) agar and enriched medium for recovery of yeast, especially *Cryptococcus neoformans*, such as Sabouraud dextrose agar (SAB), and Mycosel or mycobiotic agar, both of which inhibit bacteria and saprophytic fungi. One-half ml of BAL is inoculated on a solid medium and streaked for isolation. The streaked medium is incubated in a 30°C non-CO_2 incubator for 4 weeks. Plates are examined daily for the first week, and once a week for the remaining 3 weeks for fungal growth (Table 4.10).

Any amount of mold is typically reported to allow the physician to make the determination of clinical significance. Rare amounts of yeast are mentioned in reporting, and significant amounts of yeast are speciated, but yeast is typically an indication of upper respiratory tract contamination and rarely a causative agent in BAL specimens.

MYCOBACTERIAL CULTURE

Mycobacterium tuberculosis is highly infectious as inoculation with ≤ 10 bacilli may cause disease. Due to the risk of potential exposure to *M. tuberculosis* while performing mycobacterial culture, all manipulation of specimens, media,

Table 4.10 Significance of fungi isolated

Any amount is considered significant
- *Cryptococcus neoformans*
- *Histoplasma capsulatum*
- *Coccidioides immitis*
- *Actinomycetes* spp.
- Molds that are not considered environmental contaminates (*Aspergillus* and *Penicillium* spp. are not considered contamination unless patient is immunocompromised)

Significant amount of
- *Rhodococcus equi* in immunocompromised patients

and isolates that may cause aerosols must be conducted in biological safety level 3 environments.

Since BALs tend to be contaminated with respiratory bacteria, a decontamination/digestion step before specimen inoculation to media is necessary for the optimal recovery of AFB. Sodium hydroxide (NaOH) is toxic to bacteria and acts as an emulsifier. NaOH is combined with N-acetyl-L-cysteine (NAC) which acts as a mycolysin and dilutes the toxic NaOH. Sodium citrate is added to the process to bind heavy metals that can inactivate the NAC.

Decontamination of specimens is performed as follows: equivalent volumes of NaOH-NAC are added to no more than 10 ml of BAL in a 50 ml conical tube and vortexed. The mixture is then incubated for a maximum time of 15 minutes at room temperature, after which NaOH would begin to kill the mycobacteria. The reaction is stopped by diluting the mixture with 0.67 M phosphate buffer to the 50 ml mark of the tube and inverted to mix. To concentrate the decontaminated sample, the tube is then centrifuged at 3,000 rpm for 15 minutes in an aerosol-free sealed centrifuge container. The supernatant is then decanted into a container with disinfectant such as 10% bleach, and 1 ml of resuspension buffer or sterile isotonic saline is added to the pellet. The digested BAL sample can now be inoculated onto culture medium for incubation. Prior to incubation, the treated specimen can be examined by acid-fast staining. A portion of the digested specimen (approximately 0.5 ml) is added into an MGIT tube and 0.25 ml onto solid medium. An MGIT tube, a Lowenstein–Jensen (LJ) slant, a Middlebrook 7H11, and optional addition of selective 7H11, or Mitchison's medium may be used. LJ and 7H11 plates are incubated at 37°C without CO_2. The MGIT 960 is a fully automated instrument that uses fluorescent compounds embedded in the bottom of the MGIT tube to detect a decrease in oxygen level as the bacteria respire. Cultures are typically held for 6–8 weeks. MGIT tubes are monitored continuously by automation. Solid medium cultures are examined at 3–5 days after incubation and twice weekly for 4 weeks, and once weekly for 6–8 weeks.

Once growth is detected, contamination with other bacteria must be ruled out. In addition, there are several different techniques used to identify mycobacteria species that range from biochemical, chemiluminescent DNA probes, molecular PCR, 16S ribosomal sequencing, and MALDI. Any species of *Mycobacterium* identified is typically reported.

MOLECULAR DIAGNOSTICS

Clinical value of molecular diagnostics

Molecular diagnostics allow for rapid, specific, and sensitive detection of pathogens, commensal microorganisms, and microbial products from BAL. Diagnostic methods such as whole-genome sequencing, PCR, and real-time qPCR assays are utilized to rapidly identify respiratory pathogens by unique genes or microbial products of fungi, viruses, and bacterial species (63). These molecular testing methods give the potential for early detection of disease and an opportunity to start therapeutic treatment more rapidly; this is advantageous for organisms such as *Mycobacterium* spp., which can take weeks to culture in the laboratory. Rapid species and subspecies identification and drug resistance genotyping have become possible with PCR, PCR/MALDI-TOF, or hybridization assays. BAL proves successful in a variety of testing platforms including qPCR, MALDI-TOF mass spectrometry paired with PCR, and sequencing assays. PCR performed on BAL-extracted nucleic acid allows for early detection of viruses such as SARS-CoV-2, and fungal infections such as invasive aspergillosis, bacterial pneumonia, or *M. tuberculosis*.

PCR

Polymerase chain reaction (PCR) is used for rapid amplification of a target region of a gene. The increase in genomic data and advances in bioinformatics allows for a broader application of PCR and can be performed in single or multiplexed reactions. Traditional PCR begins with the extraction of nucleic acid from BAL fluid; the sample volume needed will vary for each extraction type. Once extracted, the nucleic acid, as little as 2 µL, is added to a PCR master mix. A typical master mix contains the following components: *Taq* polymerase, $MgCl_2$, dNTPS, buffer, primers, water, and the addition of reverse transcriptase for the synthesis of cDNA for amplification from RNA samples. When designing PCR primers, the primers should target regions of varying sizes depending on the end-point analysis performed (64). The samples undergo amplification by three cyclic reactions, which include denaturation of the double-stranded DNA to single-stranded DNA (95°C), annealing of the primers to the target sequence (primer melting temperature dependent), and extension at the 3′ terminus of the primers (72 °C). Once amplified by PCR, the samples may be further analyzed with gel electrophoresis for amplicon detection and size analysis, sequencing reactions for Sanger or whole-genome sequencing, or MALDI-TOF mass spectrometry.

PCR reactions can be multiplexed to target multiple genes from different taxa in a single reaction from BAL samples. More commercially and laboratory-developed respiratory panels are becoming available for screening of microbial species requiring no treatment before extraction of BAL. A multiplexed PCR allows for a panel screening for a variety of gene targets including the identification of pathogens, identification of genetic mutations, and drug-resistant genes. In comparison to BAL culture, PCR displays higher sensitivity in pneumonia patients undergoing antimicrobial treatment (65).

Nested PCR is used to increase the sensitivity and specificity of amplification. Nested PCR utilizes two sets of forward and reverse primer sets in a two-step PCR reaction. The first set of primers is used to create the template for the second set of primers, the oligonucleotides of the second set will anneal inside the first primer amplicon region.

Real-time PCR allows for the detection of a target by monitoring the amplification of the desired target during the PCR cycle by fluorescent probes. An advantage of this assay is that it provides quantitative results for the target pathogen amplicon. The probes fluoresce upon hybridization of the probe to the target amplicon, when fluorescence is greater than the baseline the cycle threshold value will correlate to a detected result and can be quantified. Real-time PCR assays will often show fluorescent signals in less than an hour. However, this methodology's ability for multiplex design is limited based on available fluorescent probes per reaction.

Digital droplet PCR allows for qualitative and quantitative analysis of BAL samples. This methodology separates PCR amplicons into oil-in-water droplets and eliminates the effects of PCR inhibitors (66). This assay demonstrates the potential for diagnostic advances.

VIRAL PCR

Rapid identification of viruses such as SARS-CoV-2, influenza A, influenza B, and respiratory syncytial virus can be detected from BAL using PCR-based platforms such as the real-time PCR-based Biofire FilmArray (BioFire Diagnostics, LLC, Salt Lake City, UT), RT-qPCR, or MALDI-TOF Mass Spectrometry paired with PCR MassArray Platform (Agena Biosciences, San Diego, CA). Real-time PCR assays targeting viral pneumonia focus on platforms such as the Biofire Film array, which can give not only diagnostic information but overall information about the BAL sample. The detection of SARS-CoV-2 by real-time reverse transcription (RT)-PCR methods became increasingly prevalent during the pandemic; the RT-PCR assay allows for some quantitation of viral load by CT values. For example, the TaqPath COVID-19 kit (ThermoFisher Scientific, Waltham, MA) provides data on viral load in addition to detection of SARS-CoV-2. MALDI-TOF combined PCR methods may be used to analyze combination viral panels (Table 4.11). The mass spectra results will display peaks at the corresponding mass of the unique single base extended extension probes if the target amplicon is present. The BAL sample volume needed for many PCR-based molecular tests is in the range of 200–500 µL. Other viruses commonly found in BAL samples include coronaviruses and rhinoviruses (67). Overall, real-time PCR allows for greater sensitivity of viral detection from BAL (67).

MYCOBACTERIAL PCR

The culture of both non-tuberculosis mycobacteria and *M. tuberculosis* is time-intensive and

Table 4.11 Combination MALDI-TOF and PCR method

Extract nucleic acid.

PCR with a reverse transcription one-step reaction for RNA viruses and amplification with forward and reverse primers for each viral target.

Dephosphorylate any naturally occurring nucleotides with shrimp alkaline phosphatase.

Extension reaction with terminating dideoxyribonucleoside triphosphates (ddNTPs). The highly specific extension probes will extend and terminate by a single base if the target amplicon is present.

Post the extension reaction; the samples are loaded into a MALDI-TOF platform for analysis.

tedious. Thus, rapid diagnostics for the identification and drug resistance markers provide the opportunity for earlier treatment plans. Rapid diagnostic tests such as the Cepheid GeneXpert system utilizes nested real-time PCR for the qualitative and rapid detection of *M. tuberculosis* and rifampin resistance by amplification of an 81 base pair region in IS6110. BAL samples can be added directly to a test cartridge after decontamination with NaOH and sodium citrate dihydrate followed by a digestion with NAC with same-day results. This rapid diagnostic comparison to waiting for a culture to grow which may take up to 3 weeks. Sanger sequencing of the *16S*, *hsp* (65), *erm* (41), and *rpoB* genes of mycobacteria are used for speciation and subspeciation of mycobacteria. Sanger sequencing from BAL culture of the desired mycobacterial gene begins with nucleic acid extraction. The target gene DNA is amplified by using paired forward and reverse primers for the target gene. The PCR reaction is cleaned and then labeled with fluorescent dye terminators. The final product is purified by a gel column filtration and loaded onto the genetic analyzer, which measures the fluorescence creating a sequence result. The sequence can then be analyzed with the Basic Local Alignment Search Tool (BLAST) or other appropriate genetic database for homology to determine the identification of the mycobacteria. Real-time PCR can also be utilized for

varying mycobacterial genes for rapid identification if able to identify unique, specific, and sensitive target sequences. Rapid identification and drug resistance targets for aminoglycoside and induced or acquired macrolide resistance can be rapidly identified in diagnostics by hybridization assays using both raw BAL fluid and BAL culture.

FUNGAL PCR

New molecular advancements such as the detection of the fungus *P. jirovecii* in 2.5 hours by the mitochondrial small subunit rRNA gene show the advantages of molecular testing with automation (68). Other genes such as the mitochondrial large subunit rRNA, CDC2, and multicopy major surface glycoprotein have been used for PCR detection methods of *P. jirovecii* (68). Quantitative PCR methods to detect *P. jirovecii* have demonstrated high sensitivity and specificity in comparison to other diagnostic methodologies, this is also seen in HIV-positive or low fungal load samples (69). Other advances in molecular methods include a PCR assay that has the ability not only to detect the genus *Aspergillus* but can also speciate from BAL samples and give insight to azole resistance (70, 71). A multiplex real-time PCR assay identifies different mutations associated with azole resistance in *Aspergillus fumigatus* in *CYP51A*, which azoles target (70).

Immunologic methods to detect microorganisms, their components, or specific cell responses to them

MYCOBACTERIUM TUBERCULOSIS

Enzyme-linked immunospot assays (ELISPOT) or enzyme-linked immunosorbent assays (ELISA) can be used as a rapid diagnostic tool for the identification of pulmonary *M. tuberculosis* infection from BAL samples (72). ELISPOT is an interferon-gamma (IFNγ) release assay used diagnostically to detect memory T cells that produce relatively large amounts of IFNγ in response to stimulation with relatively *M. tuberculosis*-specific antigens. BAL provides higher sensitivity of detection of IFNγ in comparison to the more traditional blood or pleural fluid samples using ELISPOT assays (72).

PNEUMOCYSTIS JIROVECII

Direct fluorescence monoclonal antibody (DFA) immunostaining aids in the diagnosis of *P. jirovecii* pneumonia with high sensitivity and specificity from BAL fluid in HIV patients (73). DFA stains have proven successful in staining pneumocystis cysts and trophic forms (74). BAL has been described as one of the most optimal sample types for the identification of *P. jirovecii* (75).

COMPONENTS OF FUNGAL ORGANISMS

Microbial products such as galactomannan and 1,3-β-D-glucan can be detected from BAL samples to help aid in the diagnosis of fungal infections such as invasive aspergillosis (IA). Molecular testing to detect these fungal biomarkers in BAL samples allows for a significant change in sensitivity in comparison to the lesser sensitive culture methods, which cause difficulty in the diagnosis of IA (76, 77). Enzyme-linked immunoassays have shown greater sensitivity as a diagnostic tool in comparison to the laboratory culture of *Aspergillus*. Platelia™ is a commercially available diagnostic sandwich ELISA for the detection of galactomannan in BAL. The optical density is read from the colorimetric assay after a monoclonal antibody targeting *Aspergillus* galactomannan is bound by a peroxidase-linked antibody and the substrate is added (78). Detection of the fungal cell wall component 1,3-β-D-glucan can assist in the detection of fungal infections.

MALDI-TOF mass spectrometry

Matrix-assisted laser desorption/ionization-time-of-flight (MALDI-TOF) mass spectrometry can be used for the rapid identification of bacteria, mycobacteria, and fungi. It can also be used for drug resistance markers and genetic mutations. PCR paired with MALDI-TOF mass spectrometry allows for specific identification by unique target amplicons which can be highly multiplexed. PCR/electrospray ionization (ESI)-mass spectrometry methods allow for the identification of pathogens that are unable to be grown in the lab (46, 12). Non-aspergillus molds can be identified by PCR/ESI-mass spectrometry, a known cause of mucormycosis from BAL samples. Methodologies such as PCR/ESI-mass spectrometry show promising

advancements with improvements in bioinformatic analysis (79).

Metagenomic next-generation sequencing

Metagenomic next-generation sequencing (mNGS) is promising as a tool in diagnosing atypical infections that are unidentifiable by current standard diagnostic tests (80, 48, 81, 82). mNGS can analyze many sample types including BAL. mNGS provides the ability to broadly test for pathogens without any information about the potential pathogens present. This can help alleviate broad-spectrum antibiotic therapies if the results yield information to start a targeted treatment plan (80, 48, 81). Typical sequencing can take up to 24 hours; however, methods using the MinION sequencer which utilize nanopore sequencing are able to detect microbial pathogens in <6 hours (80). Co-infections can also be identified by mNGS in BAL fluid collected from critically ill patient samples. mNGS has a greater sensitivity than traditional diagnostic tests for viruses, fungi, *M. tuberculosis*, non-tuberculous mycobacteria, and other atypical pathogens (82). BAL mNGS has also shown success in identifying *P. jirovecii* in confirmed pneumocystosis patients (83). Limitations of this methodology include the development of a mNGS pipeline with bioinformatic analysis capabilities.

CONCLUSION

BAL is a frequently performed procedure of low invasiveness and high patient tolerability that can be very helpful in the detection and narrowing of differential diagnoses for a variety of pulmonary processes. In addition to many standard clinical uses, there are exciting new roles for this procedure on the horizon.

In the future, it is likely that additional targeted diagnostics such as MALDI-TOF and PCR/ESI-mass spectrometry on BAL fluid will facilitate more rapid diagnosis of infectious pneumonia. Of particular interest is not only the ability to determine the etiology of infection but also to identify drug-resistant microbes. Such advances would transform the care of septic patients and improve adherence to antibiotic stewardship efforts. Additionally, genomic testing of BAL fluid may help clinicians differentiate patients with different forms of interstitial lung disease as well as stratify patients with lung nodules into different risk groups for lung cancer. While surgical lung biopsy remains the gold standard for the diagnosis of various lung diseases, less invasive diagnostic techniques will become adopted if their yield becomes significantly more accurate. With further development of specific and sensitive tests, diagnostics performed on BAL fluid may become able to rival the sensitivity and specificity of the current gold standard of surgical lung biopsy, reducing both time to diagnosis and morbidity and mortality associated with more invasive diagnostic procedures.

REFERENCES

1. Stitt HL. Bronchial aspiration and irrigation with a hypertonic solution. *J Med* 1927;5:112–17.
2. Ahmad M, Livingston DR, Golish JA, et al. The safety of outpatient transbronchial biopsy. *Chest* 1986 Sep;90(3):403–5.
3. Meyer KC, Raghu G, Baughman RP, et al. An official American Thoracic Society clinical practice guideline: The clinical utility of bronchoalveolar lavage cellular analysis in interstitial lung disease. *Am J Respir Crit Care Med* 2012 May 1;185(9):1004–14.
4. Bollmann BA, Seeliger B, Drick N, et al. Cellular analysis in bronchoalveolar lavage: Inherent limitations of current standard procedure. *Eur Respir J* 2017;49(6):1601844.
5. Baron EJ, Miller JM, Weinstein MP, et al. A guide to utilization of the microbiology laboratory for diagnosis of infectious diseases: 2013 recommendations by the Infectious Diseases Society of America (IDSA) and the American Society for Microbiology (ASM)(a). *Clin Infect Dis* 2013;57(4):e22–e121.
6. Heron M, Grutters JC, ten Dam-Molenkamp KM, et al. Bronchoalveolar lavage cell pattern from healthy human lung. *Clin Exp Immunol* 2012 Mar;167(3):523–31.
7. Fournier E, Tonnel AB, Gosset P, et al. Early neutrophil alveolitis after antigen inhalation in hypersensitivity pneumonitis. *Chest* 1985 Oct;88(4):563–6.
8. Artigas A, Castella X. *Bronchoalveolar Lavage (BAL) in Adult Respiratory Distress Syndrome (ARDS)*. Berlin, Heidelberg: Springer, 1991.
9. Nakos G, Kitsiouli EI, Tsangaris I, et al. Bronchoalveolar lavage fluid characteristics of early intermediate and late phases of ARDS: Alterations in leukocytes, proteins, PAF and surfactant components. *Intensive Care Med* 1998 Apr;24(4):296–303.
10. Smith DL, Deshazo RD. Bronchoalveolar lavage in asthma. An update and perspective. *Am Rev Respir Dis* 1993 Aug;148(2):523–32.
11. O'Donnell R, Breen D, Wilson S, et al. Inflammatory cells in the airways in COPD. *Thorax* 2006 May;61(5):448–54.
12. Davidson KR, Ha DM, Schwarz MI, et al. Bronchoalveolar lavage as a diagnostic procedure: A review of known cellular and molecular findings in various lung diseases. *J Thorac Dis* 2020;12(9):4991–5019.
13. Raghu G, Collard HR, Egan JJ, et al. An official ATS/ERS/JRS/ALAT statement: Idiopathic pulmonary fibrosis: Evidence-based guidelines for diagnosis and management. *Am J Respir Crit Care Med* 2011 Mar 15;183(6):788–824.
14. Szamosi DI, Bautista JM, Cornbleet J, et al. Clinical and laboratory institute. Body fluid analysis for cellular composition; approved guideline. CLSI document H56-A. In: Institute CaL, editor, 2006.
15. Gratama JW, Kraan J, Keeney M, et al. Clinical and laboratory institute. Enumeration of immunologically defined cell populations by flow cytometry; approved guideline-second edition. CLSI document H42. In: Institute CaLS, editor-A2, 2007.
16. Mortaz E, Gudarzi H, Tabarsi P, et al. Flow cytometry applications in the study of immunological lung disorders. *Iran J Allergy Asthma Immunol* 2015;14(1):12–8.

17. Dauber JH, Wagner M, Brunsvold S, et al. Flow cytometric analysis of lymphocyte phenotypes in bronchoalveolar lavage fluid: Comparison of a two-color technique with a standard immunoperoxidase assay. *Am J Respir Cell Mol Biol* 1992;7(5):531–41.

18. Caillaud DM, Vergnon JM, Madroszyk A, et al. Bronchoalveolar lavage in hypersensitivity pneumonitis: A series of 139 patients. *Inflamm Allergy Drug Targets* 2012 Feb;11(1):15–9.

19. Meyer KC, Soergel P. Variation of bronchoalveolar lymphocyte phenotypes with age in the physiologically normal lung. *Thorax* 1999;54(8):697–700.

20. Mund E, Christensson B, Larsson K, et al. Sex dependent differences in physiological ageing in the immune system of lower airways in healthy non-smoking volunteers: Study of lymphocyte subsets in bronchoalveolar lavage fluid and blood. *Thorax* 2001;56(6):450–55.

21. Meda BA, Buss DH, Woodruff RD, et al. Diagnosis and subclassification of primary and recurrent lymphoma. The usefulness and limitations of combined fine-needle aspiration cytomorphology and flow cytometry. *Am J Clin Pathol* 2000;113(5):688–99.

22. Song JY, Filie AC, Venzon D, et al. Flow cytometry increases the sensitivity of detection of leukemia and lymphoma cells in bronchoalveolar lavage specimens. *Cytom B* 2012;82(5):305–12.

23. Auerswald U, Barth J, Magnussen H. Value of CD-1-positive cells in bronchoalveolar lavage fluid for the diagnosis of pulmonary histiocytosis X. *Lung* 1991;169(6):305–9.

24. Welker L, Jorres RA, Costabel U, et al. Predictive value of BAL cell differentials in the diagnosis of interstitial lung diseases. *Eur Respir J* 2004 Dec;24(6):1000–6.

25. Baqir M, Vassallo R, Maldonado F, et al. Utility of bronchoscopy in pulmonary Langerhans cell histiocytosis. *J Bronchol Interv Pulmonol* 2013 Oct;20(4):309–12.

26. van Rijt LS, Kuipers H, Vos N, et al. A rapid flow cytometric method for determining the cellular composition of bronchoalveolar lavage fluid cells in mouse models of asthma. *J Immunol Methods* 2004;288(1–2):111–21.

27. Paul WE, Zhu J. How are T(H)2-type immune responses initiated and amplified? *Nat Rev Immunol* 2010;10(4):225–35.

28. Litwin V. Clinical and laboratory standards institute. Validation of assays performed by flow cytometry; approved guideline – First edition, CLSI guideline H62. In: Institute CaLS, editor, 2021.

29. Chan ED, Wilson ML, Neff TA. Pulmonary botryomycosis: Its relationship to actinomycosis and to chronic aspiration pneumonia. *Clin Pulm Med* 1996;3(2):67–71.

30. Semenzato G, Poletti V. Bronchoalveolar lavage in lung cancer. *Respiration* 1992;9:44–6.

31. Bezel P, Tischler V, Robinson C, et al. Diagnostic value of bronchoalveolar lavage for diagnosis of suspected peripheral lung cancer. *Clin Lung Cancer* 2016;17(5):e151–ee56.

32. Tomar V, Vijay N, Nuwal P, et al. Comparative study of bronchoalveolar lavage, bronchial brushing, and FNAC in diagnosing malignant neoplasms of lungs. *J Cytol* 2016;33(4):210–13.

33. Stanley MW, Henry-Stanley MJ, Gajl-Peczalska KJ, et al. Hyperplasia of type II pneumocytes in acute lung injury: Cytologic findings of sequential bronchoalveolar lavage. *Am J Clin Pathol* 1992;97(5):669–77.

34. Gulbahce HE, Baker KS, Kumar P, et al. Atypical cells in bronchoalveolar lavage specimens from bone marrow transplant recipients. A potential pitfall. *Am J Clin Pathol* 2003;120(1):101–6.

35. Murphy SL, Kochanek KD, Xu J, et al. Mortality in the United States, 2020. *NCHS Data Brief* 2021;427:1–8.

36. Ahmadinejad M, Mohammadzadeh S, Pak H, et al. Bronchoalveolar lavage of ventilator-associated pneumonia patients for antibiotic resistance and susceptibility test. *Health Sci Rep* 2022;5(1):e472.

37. Pneumonia (Ventilator-Associated [VAP] and Non-Ventilator Associated Pneumonia [PNEU]) Event. *National Healthcare Safety*

Network Patient Safety Component Manual. Centers for Disease Control and Prevention, 2022.

38. Mayhall CG. Ventiliator-associated pneumonia or not? Contemporary diagnosis. *Emerg Infect Dis* 2001;7(2):200–04.

39. Kim ES, Kim EC, Lee SM, et al. Bacterial yield from quantitative cultures of bronchoalveolar lavage fluid in patients with pneumonia on antimicrobial therapy. *Korean J Intern Med* 2012 Jun;27(2):156–62.

40. Johnson SM, Saint John BE, Dine AP. Local anesthetics as antimicrobial agents: A review. *Surg Infect (Larchmt)* 2008;9(2):205–13.

41. Begec Z, Gulhas N, Toprak HI, et al. Comparison of the antibacterial activity of lidocaine 1% versus alkalinized lidocaine *in vitro*. *Curr Ther Res Clin Exp* 2007;68(4):242–48.

42. Neuwersch S, Köstenberger M, Sorschag S, et al. Antimicrobial activity of lidocaine, bupivacaine, mepivacaine and ropivacaine on *Staphylococcus epidermidis*, *Staphylococcus aureus* and *Bacillus subtilis*. *Open Pain J* 2017;10(1):1–4.

43. Olsen KM, Peddicord TE, Campbell GD, et al. Antimicrobial effects of lidocaine in bronchoalveolar lavage fluid. *J Antimicrob Chemother* 2000;45(2):217–19.

44. Samet M, Meybodi FAA, Mokarianpour T, et al. Effect of lidocaine 2% on bacterial culture of bronchial fluid. *J Coll Phys Surg Pak* 2017;27(12):771–74.

45. Mok JH, Eom JS, Jo EJ, et al. Clinical utility of rapid pathogen identification using matrix-assisted laser desorption/ionization time-of-flight mass spectrometry in ventilated patients with pneumonia: A pilot study. *Respirology* 2016 Feb;21(2):321–8.

46. Ullberg M, Luthje P, Molling P, et al. Broad-range detection of microorganisms directly from bronchoalveolar lavage specimens by PCR/electrospray ionization-mass spectrometry. *PLOS ONE* 2017;12(1):e0170033.

47. Pendleton KM, Erb-Downward JR, Bao Y, et al. Rapid pathogen identification in bacterial pneumonia using real-time metagenomics. *Am J Respir Crit Care Med* 2017;196(12):1610–12.

48. Li Y, Sun B, Tang X, et al. Application of metagenomic next-generation sequencing for bronchoalveolar lavage diagnostics in critically ill patients. *Eur J Clin Microbiol Infect Dis* 2020;39(2):369–74.

49. Young JC, Chehoud C, Bittinger K, et al. Viral metagenomics reveal blooms of anelloviruses in the respiratory tract of lung transplant recipients. *Am J Transplant* 2015;15(1):200–09.

50. Schneeberger PHH, Prescod J, Levy L, et al. Microbiota analysis optimization for human bronchoalveolar lavage fluid. *Microbiome* 2019;7(1):141.

51. Mangels JJ, Cox ME, Lindberg LH. Methanol fixation. An alternative to heat fixation of smears before staining. *Diagn Microbiol Infect Dis* 1984;2(2):129–37.

52. Hucker GJ. A new modification and application of the Gram stain. *J Bacteriol* 1921;6(4):395–97.

53. Alderwick LJ, Harrison J, Lloyd GS, et al. The mycobacterial cell wall—Peptidoglycan and arabinogalactan. *Cold Spring Harb Perspect Med* 2015;5(8):a021113.

54. Maitra A, Munshi T, Healy J, et al. Cell wall peptidoglycan in *Mycobacterium tuberculosis*: An Achilles' heel for the TB-causing pathogen. *FEMS Microbiol Rev* 2019;43(5):548–75.

55. Percival SL, Williams DW. Mycobacterium. In: Percival SL, Yates MV, Williams DW, Chalmers RM, Gray NF, editors. *Microbiology of Waterborne Diseases: Microbiological Aspects and Risks*. Elsevier, 2014.

56. Staropoli JF, Branda JA. Cord formation in a clinical isolate of *Mycobacterium marinum*. *J Clin Microbiol* 2008;46(8):2814–16.

57. Murray PR, Baron EJ, Pfaller MA, Jorgenson JH, Yolken RH, editors. *Manual of Clinical Microbiology American Society of Microbiology*, ASM Press, 2003.

58. Grocott RG. A stain for fungi in tissue sections and smears using Gomori's methenamine-silver nitrate technic. *Am J Clin Pathol* 1955;25(8):975–79.

59. Alturkistanl HA, Tashkandi F, Mohammedsaleh ZM. Histological stains: A literature review and case study. *Glob J Health Sci* 2016;8(3):72–9.

60. Adhya AK. Grocott methenamine silver positivity in neutrophils. *J Cytol* 2019;36(3):184.

61. Zarrinfar H, Kaboli S, Dolatabadi S, et al. Rapid detection of *Candida* species in bronchoalveolar lavage fluid from patients with pulmonary symptoms. *Braz J Microbiol* 2016;47(1):172–76.

62. Aigner M, Wanner M, Kreidl P, et al. Candida in the respiratory tract potentially triggers galactomannan positivity in non-hematological patients. *Antimicrob Agents Chemother* 2019;63(6):e00138-19.

63. Graf EH, Pancholi P. Appropriate use and future directions of molecular diagnostic testing. *Curr Infect Dis Rep* 2020;22(2):5.

64. Dwivedi S, Purohit P, Misra R, et al. Diseases and molecular diagnostics: A step closer to precision medicine. *Indian J Clin Biochem* 2017;32(4):374–98.

65. Tschiedel E, Goralski A, Steinmann J, et al. Multiplex PCR of bronchoalveolar lavage fluid in children enhances the rate of pathogen detection. *BMC Pulm Med* 2019;19(1):132.

66. Cho SM, Shin S, Kim Y, et al. A novel approach for tuberculosis diagnosis using exosomal DNA and droplet digital PCR. *Clin Microbiol Infect* 2020;26(7):942.e1–42.e5.

67. Garbino J, Soccal PM, Aubert JD, et al. Respiratory viruses in bronchoalveolar lavage: A hospital-based cohort study in adults. *Thorax* 2009;64(5):399–404.

68. Liu B, Totten M, Nematollahi S, et al. Development and evaluation of a fully automated molecular assay targeting the mitochondrial small subunit rRNA gene for the detection of *Pneumocystis jirovecii* in bronchoalveolar lavage fluid specimens. *J Mol Diagn* 2020;22(12):1482–93.

69. Bateman M, Oladele R, Kolls JK. Diagnosing *Pneumocystis jirovecii* pneumonia: A review of current methods and novel approaches. *Med Mycol* 2020;58(8):1015–28.

70. Chong GL, van de Sande WW, Dingemans GJ, et al. Validation of a new Aspergillus real-time PCR assay for direct detection of Aspergillus and azole resistance of Aspergillus fumigatus on bronchoalveolar lavage fluid. *J Clin Microbiol* 2015;53(3):868–74.

71. Donnelly JP, Chen SC, Kauffman CA, et al. Revision and update of the consensus definitions of invasive fungal disease from the European Organization for Research and Treatment of Cancer and the mycoses study group education and research consortium. *Clin Infect Dis* 2020;71(6):1367–76.

72. Pang C, Wu Y, Wan C, et al. Accuracy of the bronchoalveolar lavage enzyme-linked immunospot assay for the diagnosis of pulmonary tuberculosis: A meta-analysis. *Med (Baltim)* 2016;95(12):e3183.

73. Wolfson JS, Waldron MA, Sierra LS. Blinded comparison of a direct immunofluorescent monoclonal antibody staining method and a Giemsa staining method for identification of *Pneumocystis carinii* in induced sputum and bronchoalveolar lavage specimens of patients infected with human immunodeficiency virus. *J Clin Microbiol* 1990;28(9):2136–38.

74. Thomas CF, Jr, Limper AH. Pneumocystis pneumonia. *N Engl J Med* 2004;350(24):2487–98.

75. Alshahrani MY, Alfaifi M, Ahmad I, et al. *Pneumocystis jirovecii* detection and comparison of multiple diagnostic methods with quantitative real-time PCR in patients with respiratory symptoms. *Saudi J Biol Sci* 2020;27(6):1423–27.

76. Zhang X-B, Chen G-P, Lin Q-C, et al. Bronchoalveolar lavage fluid galactomannan detection for diagnosis of invasive pulmonary aspergillosis in chronic obstructive pulmonary disease. *Med Mycol* 2013;51(7):688–95.

77. Lamoth F. Galactomannan and 1,3-β-d-Glucan testing for the diagnosis of invasive aspergillosis. *J Fungi (Basel)* 2016;2(3):22.

78. de Heer K, Gerritsen MG, Visser CE, et al. Galactomannan detection in broncho-alveolar lavage fluid for invasive aspergillosis in immunocompromised patients. *Cochrane Database Syst Rev* 2019;5(5):CD012399.

79. Krifors A, Özenci V, Ullberg M, et al. PCR with electrospray ionization-mass spectrometry on bronchoalveolar lavage for detection of invasive mold infections in hematological patients. *PLOS ONE* 2019;14(2):e0212812.

80. Gu W, Deng X, Lee M, et al. Rapid pathogen detection by metagenomic next-generation sequencing of infected body fluids. *Nat Med* 2021;27(1):115–24.

81. Gaston DC, Miller HB, Fissel JA, et al. Evaluation of metagenomic and targeted next-generation sequencing workflows for detection of respiratory pathogens from bronchoalveolar lavage fluid specimens. *J Clin Microbiol* 2022;60(7):e0052622.

82. Jin X, Li J, Shao M, et al. Improving suspected pulmonary infection diagnosis by bronchoalveolar lavage fluid metagenomic next-generation sequencing: A multicenter retrospective study. *Microbiol Spectr* 2022; Epub ahead of print.

83. Lin P, Chen Y, Su S, et al. Diagnostic value of metagenomic next-generation sequencing of bronchoalveolar lavage fluid for the diagnosis of suspected pneumonia in immunocompromised patients. *BMC Infect Dis* 2022;22(1):416.

PART 2

Using BAL as a diagnostic and/or research tool (focus on disease-related aspects)

5

Respiratory infections

VERENA SCHILDGEN, VANESSA VEDDER, MICHAEL BROCKMANN, AND OLIVER SCHILDGEN

Usually, sampling of diagnostic specimens is rather uncomplicated for the majority of respiratory infections and does not require invasive techniques, but in the case of lower respiratory tract infections, the investigation of bronchoalveolar lavage fluid (BALF) provides a valuable diagnostic tool to test for infective causes. Especially serious clinical cases requiring intensive care or extracorporeal membrane oxygenation (ECMO), may profit from BALF diagnostics.

The major advantage of BALF is that no accompanying microbiome or viriome from the upper respiratory tract is present in the diagnostic specimens, which increases the likelihood of identifying the respective causative agent or at least the major contributor to the current clinical symptoms justifying the BAL procedure. Pathogens detected in BALF include viruses, bacteria, fungi, and, rarely, parasites, which originate from the lower respiratory tract (Table 5.1).

However, pathogen detection is dependent on different factors, which among others include time of investigation as well as study period, detection methods (culture vs multiplex PCR test or targeted vs undirected), and patient cohort (immunocompromised vs immunocompetent or adults vs children).

VIRAL PATHOGENS DETECTED IN BALF

Among the most common viral pathogens detected in BALF are influenza viruses, parainfluenzaviruses (PIV), rhino- and enteroviruses, respiratory syncytial viruses (RSV), human metapneumoviruses (HMPV), human coronaviruses (229E, NL63, OC43, HKU-1, SARS-CoV-2), adenoviruses, and human bocaviruses (HBoV), all of which have been shown to infect respiratory tissues and to replicate in the upper and lower respiratory tract. However, opportunistic and rare pathogens may also play a serious role and should be taken into account for differential diagnostics depending on the clinical course.

To this group belongs the MERS-coronavirus, which is typically transferred from camels to humans (1) but may also be transferred less frequently from human to human (2, 3). Further examples are human herpesviruses (4) including cytomegalovirus (CMV) and varicella zoster virus (VZV), which may cause life-threatening pneumonia in some patient groups such as immunocompromised patients or pregnant women, but also the quasi-ubiquitous viruses HSV-1 (herpes simplex virus) (5, 6) and HHV-6 (human herpes

DOI: 10.1201/9781003146834-7

Table 5.1 Overview of recent clinical studies dealing with the detection of pathogens in the BALF

Pathogen (≤3% detection rate)			Cohort	
Viral	Bacterial	Fungal	(no. of patients)	Reference
HSV1, Influenza, RV, PIV	*S. maltophilia*	*A. fumigatus*	Patients with acute leukemia ≥18 y (88)	Ghandili et al. (2022) (43)
CMV	*M. tuberculosis*	*P. jirovecii*	HIV-positive patients ≥10 y (1768)	Chen et al. (2022) (54)
RSV	*S. pneumoniae, K. pneumoniae, E. coli, P. aeruginosa*	*Aspergillus* spp., *P. jirovecii*	Patients with hematological malignancies ≥18 y (353)	Zak et al. (2020) (36)
HADV, HRV, HRSV, HPIV	*M. pneumoniae, S. pneumoniae, H. influenzae, M. catarrhalis*	No data	Hospitalized children ≤14 y (573)	Wang et al. (2021) (55)
No data	*K. pneumoniae*	*C. albicans, C. tropicalis*	Hospitalized patients ≥16 y (153)	Singh et al. (2018) (56)
No data	*S. aureus, S. pneumoniae, H. influenzae, E. coli*	*A. fumigatus*	Patients ≤25y (70)	Tschiedel et al. (2019) (18)
-	*S. aureus, H. influenzae, P. aeruginosa*	-	Children with CF ≤7 y (215)	Gangell et al. (2011) (57)
Rhinovirus	+ No details provided	+ No details provided	Patients with serious acute respiratory illness (mean age 55 ± 15 y) (283)	Sumino et al. (2010) (58)
HSV-1, CMV, EBV, HHV-6	*Streptococcus* spp., *Staphylococcus* spp.	*P. jirovecii, Candida* sp., *Aspergillus* sp.	Adults with viral test(s) performed ≥18 y (212)	Jouneau et al. (2013) (59)
HCoV, HRV, PIV, CMV	+ No details provided	*P. jirovecii*	Adult immunocompromised patients (mean age 52 y) (299)	Garbino et al. (2009) (60)
Influenza, HMPV, RV/ Entero, RSV	+ No details provided	No data	Adult patients with acute respiratory distress ≥18 y (276)	Bouzid et al. (2023) (61)
No data	*S. pneumoniae, H. influenzae, M. catarrhalis*	No data	Children with chronic LRTI 0.5–6 y (122)	Montaner et al. (2018) (15)

(*Continued*)

Table 5.1 (Continued)

Parasites	Cohort (no. of patients)	Reference
Strongyloides stercoralis	1	Kumar et al. (2022) (62)
Paragonimus westermani	1	Meehan et al. (2002) (63)
Lophomonas sp.	5	Failoc-Rojas et al. (2020) (64)
Tetratrichomonas spp., *Trichomonas* tenax	10 (out of 115)	Lin et al. (2019) (65)
Schistosoma mansoni	1	Abdulla et al. (1999) (66)
Toxoplasma gondii	3	Jacobs et al. (1991) (67)

No data = information not available from reference
- = below 3%

virus)(7) may be associated with serious clinical courses such as pneumomediastinum or pneumothorax (8).

Whereas the majority of typical respiratory viruses, with the exception of HBoV, do not persist and a positive PCR and/or cell culture result indicates an acute infection, the ability of herpesviruses to persist hampers the discrimination between an active replicative infection or a persistence-induced "colonization." As high viral loads are more likely to be observed in cases in which herpesviruses are the causative agents, the viral load quantification may give an indication to what extent the infection is caused by the respective virus. Nevertheless, an accompanying serological test should be performed for confirmation (7).

Moreover, it has to be noted that any quantification out of BALFs remains hard to standardize. On the one hand, the BAL procedure itself determines the quantification, as the instilled as well as the recovered liquid volume directly influence the maximal concentration. On the other hand, the comparability of viral loads from different institutions is strongly dependent on the respective level of BAL sampling protocols standardization, not yet taking into account patient-specific factors. Furthermore, quantification methods, type of viral nucleic acid extraction, and equipment technology may influence the diagnostic outcome.

As the microbiological and virological analysis of BALF normally only takes place in critically ill patients, prompt diagnostics are required, which are supported by multiplexing techniques that enable rapid analysis of the most relevant obligate and facultative respiratory pathogens. Assays that could be used with BALF, either as certified for this specimen type or due to published data using BALF as a specimen, are the Respi-/MeningoFinder 2Smart assays (Pathofinder, Maastricht, the Netherlands), the QiaStat Respiratory Assay (Qiagen, Hilden, Germany), the BioFire multiplex assay (BioMerieux, Lyon, France), or the Anyplex™ II RV 16 kit (Seegene, Inc., Seoul, South Korea), to give some examples (9–13). In consideration of the European in vitro diagnostic medical devices regulations (IVDR), which were released by the European Commission in 2017 and applied since 2022, BALF specimens require an in-house validation in case their usage is not explicitly stated in the vendors' validation protocols.

In the context of multiplexing technologies, it is important to note that with their increasing use, the reports of multiple infections in critically ill patients also increased, which requires defined cut-off values to distinguish between persistence or active co- and superinfections and to identify the leading pathogen that is most likely responsible for the respective clinical course.

BACTERIAL PATHOGENS DETECTED IN THE BALF

In many infections of the lower respiratory tract bacteria are the leading pathogens. These include but are not limited to typical respiratory bacteria such as *Haemophilus influenzae*, *Legionella pneumoniae*, *Chlamydia pneumophila*, *Staphylococcus* spp., and *Streptococcus* spp. Additionally, *Mycoplasma* spp., *Mycobacterium tuberculosis*, and mycobacteria other than tuberculosis (MOTT) are recurrently detected in BALF.

The majority of bacterial-induced cases are already suspected to cause the clinical course due to radiological findings of a typical pneumonia, which rarely leads to BALF analyses. For this reason, in BALF, bacteria are frequently observed as co-pathogens of viral infections (14), but also co-detection of multiple bacteria are common when molecular tests are used (15–17). According to multiplex PCR assays used in clinical virology, nucleic acid detection assays are, meanwhile, also able to identify the most common causes of bacterial pneumonia (16). Several studies suggest that bacterial multiplex PCR assays provide faster results along with a higher pathogen detection rate in patients undergoing BAL for suspicion of pulmonary infection than conventional culture (18–20). On the one hand, these molecular tests decrease the likelihood of missing relevant organisms, especially in the case of so far unculturable pathogens or if it is not possible to isolate atypical bacterial pathogens and viruses due to limited resources. On the other hand, the increased analytic sensitivity may complicate clinical decision-making, as non-viable organisms are also detected. For this reason, in most cases the gold standard for diagnostics of bacterial infections still remains culturing, although there are significant disadvantages as the need for trained manpower for this labor-intensive process, limited sensitivity based on sample quality, and time periods of days to weeks to confirm the diagnosis.

FUNGAL AND PARASITIC PATHOGENS IN THE BALF

The most relevant example of an unculturable pathogen in routine diagnostics is *P. jirovecii*, which was initially classified as a parasite, but due to molecular investigations was, post-millennium, reclassified as a fungus. This organism is both a pathogen, especially in the immunosuppressed patient and less frequently in immunocompetent individuals, and also a facultative bystander. *P. jirovecii* is either identified microscopically or more frequently by PCR. In this case high gene copy numbers may be indicative of true infections, while lower gene copy numbers most likely suggest asymptomatic colonization in the immunocompetent host (21, 22). While further fungi may also act as pathogens and could be detected in the BALF by culturing, these infections are rather rare in industrialized countries except for *Aspergillus* infections, which are frequently observed in critically ill patients (23). The *Aspergillus* diagnostics out of BALF specimens may include a Galactomannan-ELISA, which is validated for blood and serum, but which also works properly for BALF (24).

Although several parasites may elicit lung diseases as a result of transient passage in the lung, such infections are rarely identified (Table 5.1). In industrialized countries worm infections mainly affect individuals who perform outdoor activities in contact with wildlife (e.g., hunting), have extensive contact with farm or domestic animals, or homeless people often accompanied by drug abuse (25–30). Nevertheless, certain helminth infections such as strongyloidiasis may be underdiagnosed in non-endemic areas due to the presence of asymptomatic individuals, the lack of awareness of the disease, and the poor sensitivity of diagnostic methods, although the respective larvae can be identified in BALF (31). Infection by protozoans is a rare condition, which is mostly associated with the status of immunosuppression and/or poor hygiene conditions in underdeveloped countries. Considering increasing globalization and travel activity, it becomes more and more important to consider parasitic infections as differential diagnosis of lung diseases even in non-endemic regions.

COLONIZATION OR INFECTION?

For some pathogens, there is an established differentiation between a true infection and an asymptomatic colonization. With regard to *P. jirovecii*, Morris and Norris define colonization as an occasionally detected condition during routine testing such as immunohistochemical staining, that "in contrast to Pneumocystis infection occurs in persons without signs or symptoms of acute pneumonia" (32). Thereby Morris and Norris remain vague to what extent a quantification of gene or genome copies of *Pneumocystis* is a suitable tool to discriminate between infection and colonization, as the majority of quantitative diagnostic assays for *P. jirovecii* amplifies a multicopy gene impeding proper quantification and leading to up to one log-step deviation (32). This diagnostic blurring is extended by the fact that scientists have found evidence that several circulating *P. jirovecii* strains may have different genetic and epigenetic backgrounds with alterations also related to the copy number of the multicopy genes (33, 34). Nevertheless, at least in immunocompromised patients, a discrimination between infection and colonization is accepted, although cut-off values differ between 340 multicopy surface gene copies per mL BALF (35) and $\geq$1,450 copies/mL of a not-further-specified gene as a threshold of colonization and infection (36). In contrast, immunocompetent patients with rather mild clinical infections characterized by chronic cough without pneumonia often show low *P. jirovecii* titers that according to these earlier definitions would have been assessed as a colonization (37).

Other common pathogens that can also colonize the patients and may be detected in the BALF are *Candida* spp. (38) and *Haemophilus influenzae* (39) with colonization rates of up to 25% and 75% respectively, depending on study cohorts.

Regarding viral pathogens, it is more difficult to differentiate between colonization and infection, as some viruses that infect the lung or may replicate in the airways are able to establish a productive or unproductive persistent infection. While Zak and coworkers define certain thresholds for HSV and CMV (36), this does not necessarily reflect any internationally accepted consensus but reveals a problematic issue in multi-pathogen detections.

As many pathogens discussed here are known causative agents of respiratory disease, in the case of multi-pathogen infection the question arises if there is a leading pathogen or if the combination of all present pathogens, independent of their respective pathogenicity, is responsible for the respective clinical course.

Stram and coworkers analyzed the viral genome copy number load of HSV-1 and the number of infectious HSV-1 particles in the lower respiratory tract of organ transplant recipients and critically ill patients (40). They observed that the clinical outcome in HSV-1 positive patients was worse compared to HSV-1 negative individuals if viral loads exceed 1.3×10^3 copies/mL BALF (40). This finding is confirmed by the study of den Brink and colleagues, who also observed a higher mortality in HSV-1 positive patients suffering from critical illness conditions, but without discriminating between colonization and infection (41). Nevertheless, it should be noted, that others work with viral load thresholds of $\geq$10^5 copies/mL of BALF to define infection versus lower respiratory tract colonization, as they observed worse clinical outcomes above this cut-off (36, 42).

While the detection of HSV in the BALF may have an impact on the drug regimen and may lead to a novel medication as reported by Ghandili et al. (43), these discrepant results regarding cut-off thresholds show that a true discrimination between colonization and infection is not possible for persisting viruses that in case of herpesviruses is lifelong and may alter between phases of low and high-level active replication, or silent persistence. For CMV, another herpesvirus, these cut-off values appear to be more established, as several studies identified 500 IU/mL as the threshold with the highest possible likelihood discriminate between persistence and active replication leading to life-threatening pneumonia (44, 45).

There is also a lack of consensus regarding the bacterial load discriminating true infection or colonization of the lower airways or contamination, respectively, on cut-off values to differentiate infection from upper respiratory tract contamination when culturing BALFs. The cut-off range varies between 10^5 CFU/mL (46, 47), 10^4 CFU/mL (17), and 10^3 CFU/mL (19) taking into account that thresholds depend on single or multiple pathogen detection or even on the identification of specific organisms regardless of colony counts (15, 19).

CYTOLOGICAL FEATURES OF PATHOGEN-POSITIVE BALS

To date there are limited data available on differential cytology of BALF from patients with infectious disease and it is rather assumed than proven that bacterial infections go ahead with increased macrophage and granulocyte counts while viral infections are associated with increased levels of T-lymphocytes.

Differential cytology of BALF specimens in general starts with a microscopic analysis of cytospin samples stained with classical histological techniques like May–Grünwald–Giemsa stain, hematoxylin-eosin stain, periodic acid–Schiff reaction, and Prussian blue or Turnbull staining. These stainings enable the differentiation of BALF-associated cells into macrophages, eosinophilic granulocytes, neutrophilic granulocytes, lymphocytes, and plasma/mast cells. Further differentiation is performed at threshold minima of 6% lymphocytes in smoking and 10–15% lymphocytes in non-smoking patients as loosely established cut-off values in the current literature and requires additional immuno-staining or flow cytometry methods. Guidelines that are still in use are the guidelines from the American Thoracic Society (48) and the *BAL Atlas* by Costabel (49). Costabel extracted the threshold data from several earlier publications and found that the cell populations in BALs from otherwise healthy probands consist of 80% macrophages, up to 15% lymphocytes, up to 3% neutrophilic cells, up to 0.5% of eosinophilic cells, and up to 0.5% of mast cells. In contrast, smokers have elevated macrophage levels and lower lymphocyte counts despite normal to high overall cell counts. According to his findings the lymphocyte distribution of otherwise healthy non-smokers (ns) vs smokers (s) differs regarding CD4+-cells (40–70% vs 20–50%), CD8+-cells (20–40% vs 30–70%), the resulting T4/T8 ratio (1.1–3.5 vs 0.5–1.5), CD1a+ Langerhans cells (<3% vs <4%), and CD57+-cells (2–14% vs 1–11%). In otherwise healthy individuals the proportion of B-cells (<4%), CD3+ (63–83%), and activated T-cells (<5%) seems to be independent of smoking status.

In case of neutrophils, mast cells, and the overall lymphocyte cell count the guidelines of the American Thoracic Society match with the threshold values proposed by Costabel, whereas there are slight differences regarding the proportion of macrophages (>85%), eosinophils (≤1%) and the T4/T8 ratio (0.9–2.5) in normal/healthy adult non-smokers (48). All cell counts were measured by the cytocentrifuge method.

In order to add more details, which could supplement the BALF differential cytology, we analyzed our own patient cohort and extracted BALF data of patients with a proven bacterial, viral, or fungal-associated disease. Out of 3,628 BALFs collected between 2017 to 2020, we identified 442 patients with at least one pathogen detected in the BALF and compared the respective staining-based cell profiles (Figure 5.1).

Classical stainings revealed no significant differences with regard to the total macrophage counts, except that all types of infections reduce the overall cell count compared to the standard reference range defined by Costabel (49). Differences were observed between smokers (s) and non-smokers (ns), but only the direct comparison of viral vs fungal infection and viral vs multiple infections displayed a statistically significant difference for the overall macrophage count (Table 5.2). Lymphocyte and neutrophilic granulocyte counts are elevated during infection regarding the reference values, but also do not differ among the pathogens. Plasma cells are occasionally observed independent of infection cause and other cell types are also not observed.

A more differentiated cell profile was observed by flow cytometry (Figure 5.2) analyzing 212 of the aforementioned 442 specimens due to elevated lymphocyte counts. Nevertheless, also in

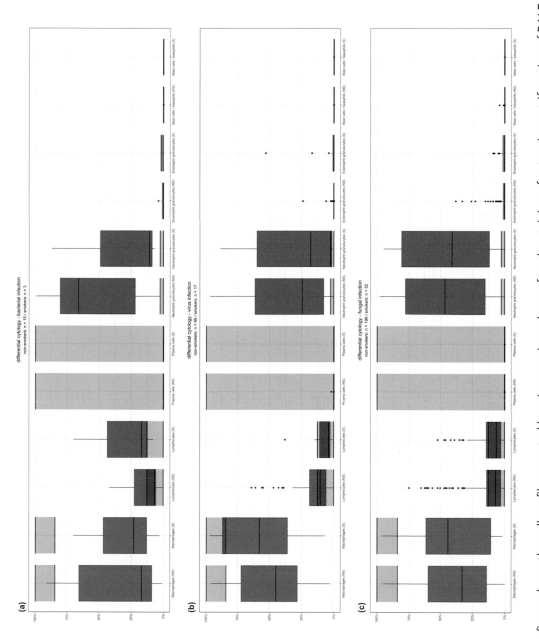

Figure 5.1 The figure shows the cell profiles counted by microscopic analyses after the staining of cytospin centrifugation of BALFs. Panel (a) shows the cohort infected with bacteria, panel (b) represents viral infection, and panel (c) fungal infections. Grey columns represent the reference values as defined by Costabel (49). Smokers (S) and non-smokers (NS) are compared side by side.

Table 5.2 The table displays the differences between several types of infection (B: bacterial; V: viral; F: fungal; M: multiple pathogens) in the cell patterns in BALF counted by microscopic analyses after cytospin centrifugation staining. The p values represent the result obtained by a 2-sides Student's T-test

Cells	Differential cytology		Macrophages		Lymphocytes		Plasma cells		Neutrophil granulocytes		Eosinophil granulocytes		Mast cells / basophils	
	n (B)	n (V)	B	V	B	V	B	V	B	V	B	V	B	V
Bacterial infection / virus infection	18	83	35,17 ± 30.97 p = 0.06	48,84 ± 27.29	17.12 ± 17.13 p = 0.47	14.28 ± 14.55	0.01 ± 0.02 p = 0.67	0.03 ± 0.22	49.72 ± 34.11 p = 0.07	34.70 ± 30.84	0.82 ± 1.19 p = 0.64	1.55 ± 6.59	0.01 ± 0.03 p = 0.72	0.01 ± 0.03
	n (B)	n (F)	B	F	B	F	B	F	B	F	B	F	B	F
Bacterial infection / fungal infection	18	249	35.17 ± 30.97 p = 0.59	38.88 ± 28.00	17.12 ± 17.13 p = 0.20	12.47 ± 14.54	0.01 ± 0.02 p = 0.99	0.01 ± 0.02	49.72 ± 34.11 p = 0.65	46,07 ± 32.70	0.82 ± 1.19 p = 0.44	1.72 ± 4.96	0.01 ± 0.03 p = 0.72	0.03 ± 0.26
	n (V)	n (F)	V	F	V	F	V	F	V	F	V	F	V	F
Virus infection / fungal infection	83	249	48.84 ± 27.29 P = 0.01	38.88 ± 28.00	14.28 ± 14.55 p = 0.33	12.47 ± 14.54	0.03 ± 0.22 P = 0.12	0.01 ± 0.02	34.70 ± 30.84 P = 0.01	46.07 ± 32.70	1.55 ± 6.59 P = 0.80	1.72 ± 4.96	0.01 ± 0.03 P = 0.40	0.03 ± 0.26
	n (B)	n (M)	B	M	B	M	B	M	B	M	B	M	B	M
Bacterial infection / multiple infections	18	36	35.17 ± 30.97 p = 0.67	31.56 ± 28.39	17.12 ± 17.13 p = 0.97	17.34 ± 19.96	0.01 ± 0.02 p = 0.16	0.00 ± 0.00	49.72 ± 34.11 p = 0.97	49.28 ± 36.26	0.82 ± 1.19 p = 0.61	1.86 ±8.46	0.01 ± 0.03 p = 0.75	0.01 ± 0.03
	n (V)	n (M)	V	M	V	M	V	M	V	M	V	M	V	M
Virus infection / multiple infections	83	36	48.84 ± 27.29 p = 0.00	31.56 ± 28.39	14.28 ± 14.55 p = 0.35	17.34 ± 19.96	0.03 ± 0.22 p = 0.45	0.00 ± 0.00	34.70 ± 30.84 p = 0.03	49.28 ± 36.26	1.55 ± 6.59 p = 0.83	1.86 ± 8.46	0.01 ± 0.03 p = 0.99	0.01 ± 0.03
	n (F)	n (M)	F	M	F	M	F	M	F	M	F	M	F	M
Fungal infection / multiple infections	249	36	38.88 ± 28.00 p = 0.14	31.56 ± 28.39	12.47 ± 14.54 p = 0.08	17.34 ± 19.96	0.01 ± 0.02 p = 0.15	0.00 ± 0.00	46.07 ± 32.70 p = 0.59	49.28 ± 36.26	1.72 ± 4.96 p = 0.89	1.86 ± 8.46	0.03 ± 0.26 p = 0.57	0.01 ± 0.03

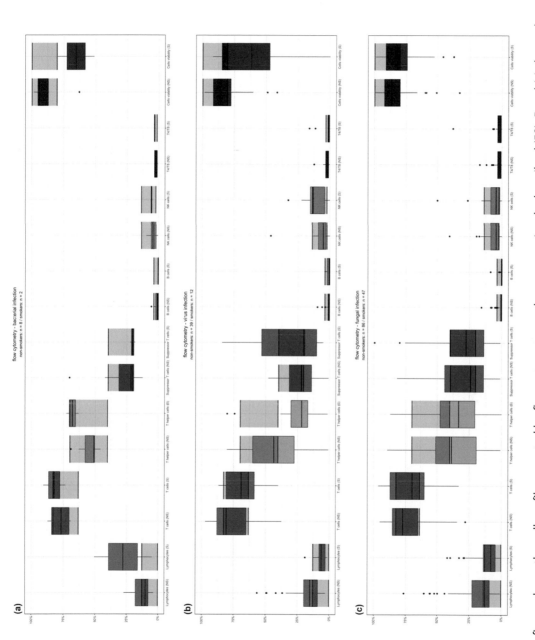

Figure 5.2 The figure shows the cell profiles counted by flow cytometry analyses as previously described (53). Panel (a) shows the cohort infected with bacteria, panel (b) represents viral infection, and panel (c) fungal infections. Grey columns represent the reference values as defined by Costabel (49). Smokers (S) and non-smokers (NS) are compared side by side.

Table 5.3 The table displays the differences between several types of infection (B: bacterial; V: viral; F: fungal; M: multiple pathogens) in the cell patterns in BALF counted flow cytometry analyses as previously described (53). The p values represent the result obtained by a 2-sides Student's T-test

Cells	Flow cytometry		Lymphocytes		T-cells		T-helper cells		Suppressor T-cells		B-cells		NK-cells		T4/T8		Cells viability	
	n(B)	n(V)	B	V	B	V	B	V	B	V	B	V	B	V	B	V	B	V
Bacterial infection / virus infection	10	51	15.59 ±14.37 p=1.00	15.56 ±12.64	78.13 ±7.89 p=0.37	73.52 ±15.73	57.26 ±9.11 p=0.03	39.99 ±23.32	27.47 ±16.94 p=0.64	24.73 ±16.83	1.55 ±1.83 p=0.65	1.27 ±1.77	5.02 ±2.68 p=0.28	7.91 ±8.18	2.59 ±1.03 p=0.98	2.58 ±3.07	84.60 ±15.78 p=0.26	77.13 ±19.48
	n(B)	n(F)	B	F	B	F	B	F	B	F	B	F	B	F	B	F	B	F
Bacterial infection / fungal infection	10	133	15.59 ±14.37 p=0.89	16.21 ±13.61	78.13 ±7.89 p=0.34	73.49 ±15.12	57.26 ±9.11 p=0.00	35.75 ±22.10	27.47 ±16.94 p=0.60	31.18 ±21.96	1.55 ±1.83 p=0.37	0.94 ±2.10	5.02 ±2.68 p=0.46	6.65 ±6.85	2.59 ±1.03 p=0.90	2.44 ±3.93	84.60 ±15.78 p=0.67	82.74 ±12.85
	n(V)	n(F)	V	F	V	F	V	F	V	F	V	F	V	F	V	F	V	F
Virus infection / fungal infection	51	133	15.56 ±12.64 p=0.77	16.21 ±13.61	73.52 ±15.73 p=0.99	73.49 ±15.12	39.99 ±23.32 p=0.25	35.75 ±22.10	24.73 ±16.83 p=0.06	31.18 ±21.96	1.27 ±1.77 p=0.32	0.94 ±2.10	7.91 ±8.18 p=0.29	6.65 ±6.85	2.58 ±3.07 p=0.83	2.44 ±3.93	77.13 ±19.48 p=0.02	82.74 ±12.85
	n(B)	n(M)	B	M	B	M	B	M	B	M	B	M	B	M	B	M	B	M
Bacterial infection / multiple infections	10	19	15.59 ±14.37 p=0.35	20.33 ±12.04	78.13 ±7.89 p=0.62	75.10 ±17.84	57.26 ±9.11 p=0.00	33.10 ±19.13	27.47 ±16.94 p=0.59	32.15 ±24.38	1.55 ±1.83 p=0.07	0.65 ±0.75	5.02 ±2.68 p=0.62	7.02 ±12.47	2.59 ±1.03 p=0.53	2.16 ±2.00	84.60 ±15.78 p=0.99	84.53 ±12.46
	n(V)	n(M)	V	M	V	M	V	M	V	M	V	M	V	M	V	M	V	M
Virus infection / multiple infections	51	19	15.56 ±12.64 p=0.16	20.33 ±12.04	73.52 ±15.73 p=0.72	75.10 ±17.84	39.99 ±23.32 p=0.25	33.10 ±19.13	24.73 ±16.83 p=0.15	32.15 ±24.38	1.27 ±1.77 p=0.15	0.65 ±0.75	7.91 ±8.18 p=0.73	7.02 ±12.47	2.58 ±3.07 p=0.58	2.16 ±2.00	77.13 ±19.48 p=0.13	84.53 ±12.46
	n(F)	n(M)	F	M	F	M	F	M	F	M	F	M	F	M	F	M	F	M
Fungal infection / multiple infections	133	19	16.21 ±13.61 p=0.21	20.33 ±12.04	73.49 ±15.12 p=0.67	75.10 ±17.84	35.75 ±22.10 p=0.62	33.10 ±19.13	31.18 ±21.96 p=0.86	32.15 ±24.38	0.94 ±2.10 p=0.56	0.65 ±0.75	6.65 ±6.85 p=0.85	7.02 ±12.47	2.44 ±3.93 p=0.76	2.16 ±2.00	82.74 ±12.85 p=0.57	84.53 ±12.46

these analyses, only a few statistically significant cell pattern differences can be observed among the different pathogens identified in the BALF. These differences, as shown in Table 5.3 and Figure 5.2, are mainly restricted to the different counts of T-cells and T-helper cells and are not group spanning but limited to some subgroups. In conclusion, while infectious diseases cause a higher overall lymphocyte count in the BALF compared to healthy individuals, no obvious differences can be observed only on the basis of cytological and flow cytometry investigations. Consequently, any suspected infection must be properly diagnosed by usage of microbiological and virological measures such as culturing and nucleic acid testing.

OTHER ASPECTS OF PATHOGEN DETECTION IN BALF

Occasionally, a comprehensive analysis of a BALF's microbiome may be useful, especially in chronic infections and chronic clinical courses to identify the causative agent.

In this context, protracted bacterial bronchitis in Italian children could be traced back to moderate bacterial loads with pathogens such as *Haemophilus influenzae, Streptococcus pneumoniae*, and *Moraxella catarrhalis* (50).

Additionally, a further systematic review study gave rise to the hypothesis that the lung microbiome is altered in patients with idiopathic pulmonary fibrosis in comparison to patients without fibrosis (51). Although the authors conclude that the observed correlations between pathogens (e.g., HSV) and fibroses do "not necessarily entail causation," the causal link appears highly likely. Furthermore, a case report published by our group has shown that chronic cough could be associated with a persistent HBoV infection, which shows active (symptomatic) and replication inactive (asymptomatic) phases during the clinical course, an observation that was only possible by proper usage of BAL and BALF as diagnostic tools (52).

Finally, the topic of the usage of BALF diagnostics in case of serious COVID-19 also has to be discussed. Despite a plethora of literature on COVID-19 in general, there are still limited data on the cytological profile of the BALF fluid in this disease. To date, it still appears that the cytological analysis alone is not specific enough to differentiate between COVID-19 and any other disease on cytological profiles, thus again a molecular analysis in the sense of a nucleic acid testing is still required (53).

REFERENCES

1. de Wit E, van Doremalen N, Falzarano D, Munster VJ. SARS and MERS: Recent insights into emerging coronaviruses. *Nature Reviews in Microbiology.* 2016;14(8):523–34.
2. Cho SY, Kang JM, Ha YE, Park GE, Lee JY, Ko JH, et al. MERS-CoV outbreak following a single patient exposure in an emergency room in South Korea: An epidemiological outbreak study. *Lancet.* 2016;388(10048):994–1001.
3. Bin SY, Heo JY, Song MS, Lee J, Kim EH, Park SJ, et al. Environmental contamination and viral shedding in MERS patients during MERS-CoV outbreak in South Korea. *Clinical Infectious Diseases: An Official Publication of the Infectious Diseases Society of America.* 2016;62(6):755–60.
4. Clementi N, Ghosh S, De Santis M, Castelli M, Criscuolo E, Zanoni I, et al. Viral respiratory pathogens and lung injury. *Clinical Microbiology Reviews.* 2021;34(3).
5. Giacobbe DR, Di Bella S, Dettori S, Brucci G, Zerbato V, Pol R, et al. Reactivation of herpes simplex virus Type 1 (HSV-1) detected on bronchoalveolar lavage fluid (BALF) samples in critically ill COVID-19 patients undergoing invasive mechanical ventilation: Preliminary results from two Italian centers. *Microorganisms.* 2022;10(2).
6. Luzzati R, D'Agaro P, Busca A, Maurel C, Martellani F, Rosin C, et al. Herpes simplex virus (HSV) pneumonia in the non-ventilated immunocompromised host: Burden and predictors. *The Journal of Infection.* 2019;78(2):127–33.
7. Bauer CC, Jaksch P, Aberle SW, Haber H, Lang G, Klepetko W, et al. Relationship between cytomegalovirus DNA load in

epithelial lining fluid and plasma of lung transplant recipients and analysis of coinfection with Epstein-Barr virus and human herpesvirus 6 in the lung compartment. *Journal of Clinical Microbiology.* 2007;45(2):324–8.

8. Lopez-Rivera F, Colon Rivera X, Gonzalez Monroig HA, Garcia Puebla J. Pneumomediastinum and pneumothorax associated with herpes simplex virus (HSV) pneumonia. *The American Journal of Case Reports.* 2018;19:109–13.

9. Babady NE. The FilmArray(R) respiratory panel: An automated, broadly multiplexed molecular test for the rapid and accurate detection of respiratory pathogens. *Expert Review of Molecular Diagnostics.* 2013;13(8):779–88.

10. Ramanan P, Bryson AL, Binnicker MJ, Pritt BS, Patel R. Syndromic panel-based testing in clinical microbiology. *Clinical Microbiology Reviews.* 2018;31(1).

11. Zhang N, Wang L, Deng X, Liang R, Su M, He C, et al. Recent advances in the detection of respiratory virus infection in humans. *Journal of Medical Virology.* 2020;92(4):408–17.

12. Huang HS, Tsai CL, Chang J, Hsu TC, Lin S, Lee CC. Multiplex PCR system for the rapid diagnosis of respiratory virus infection: Systematic review and meta-analysis. *Clinical Microbiology and Infection: The Official Publication of the European Society of Clinical Microbiology and Infectious Diseases.* 2018;24(10):1055–63.

13. Mayer LM, Kahlert C, Rassouli F, Vernazza P, Albrich WC. Impact of viral multiplex real-time PCR on management of respiratory tract infection: A retrospective cohort study. *Pneumonia.* 2017;9:4.

14. Klein EY, Monteforte B, Gupta A, Jiang W, May L, Hsieh YH, et al. The frequency of influenza and bacterial coinfection: A systematic review and meta-analysis. *Influenza and Other Respiratory Viruses.* 2016;10(5):394–403.

15. Escribano Montaner A, Garcia de Lomas J, Villa Asensi JR, Asensio de la Cruz O, de la Serna Blazquez O, Santiago Burruchaga M, et al. Bacteria from bronchoalveolar lavage fluid from children with suspected chronic lower respiratory tract infection: Results from a multi-center, cross-sectional study in Spain. *European Journal of Pediatrics.* 2018;177(2):181–92.

16. Hanson KE, Azar MM, Banerjee R, Chou A, Colgrove RC, Ginocchio CC, et al. Molecular testing for acute respiratory tract infections: Clinical and diagnostic recommendations from the IDSA's diagnostics committee. *Clinical Infectious Diseases: An Official Publication of the Infectious Diseases Society of America.* 2020;71(10):2744–51.

17. Hedberg P, Johansson N, Ternhag A, Abdel-Halim L, Hedlund J, Naucler P. Bacterial co-infections in community-acquired pneumonia caused by SARS-CoV-2, influenza virus and respiratory syncytial virus. *BMC Infectious Diseases.* 2022;22(1):108.

18. Tschiedel E, Goralski A, Steinmann J, Rath PM, Olivier M, Mellies U, et al. Multiplex PCR of bronchoalveolar lavage fluid in children enhances the rate of pathogen detection. *BMC Pulmonary Medicine.* 2019;19(1):132.

19. Salina A, Schumann DM, Franchetti L, Jahn K, Purkabiri K, Muller R, et al. Multiplex bacterial PCR in the bronchoalveolar lavage fluid of non-intubated patients with suspected pulmonary infection: A quasi-experimental study. *ERJ Open Research.* 2022;8(2).

20. Baudel JL, Tankovic J, Dahoumane R, Carrat F, Galbois A, Ait-Oufella H, et al. Multiplex PCR performed of bronchoalveolar lavage fluid increases pathogen identification rate in critically ill patients with pneumonia: A pilot study. *Annals of Intensive Care.* 2014;4:35.

21. White PL, Backx M, Barnes RA. Diagnosis and management of *Pneumocystis jirovecii* infection. *Expert Review of Anti-Infective Therapy.* 2017;15(5):435–47.

22. Fan LC, Lu HW, Cheng KB, Li HP, Xu JF. Evaluation of PCR in bronchoalveolar lavage fluid for diagnosis of *Pneumocystis*

jirovecii pneumonia: A bivariate meta-analysis and systematic review. *PLOS ONE.* 2013;8(9):e73099.

23. Vivek KU, Kumar N. Microbiological profile of bronchoalveolar lavage fluid in patients with chronic respiratory diseases: A tertiary care hospital study. *International Journal of Medical Research and Review.* 2016;4(3):330–7.

24. Bassetti M, Giacobbe DR, Grecchi C, Rebuffi C, Zuccaro V, Scudeller L, et al. Performance of existing definitions and tests for the diagnosis of invasive aspergillosis in critically ill, adult patients: A systematic review with qualitative evidence synthesis. *The Journal of Infection.* 2020;81(1):131–46.

25. Kaduszkiewicz H, Bochon B, van den Bussche H, Hansmann-Wiest J, van der Leeden C. The medical treatment of homeless people. *Deutsches Arzteblatt International.* 2017;114(40):673–9.

26. Juckett G. Common intestinal helminths. *American Family Physician.* 1995;52(7):2039–48, 2051–2.

27. Echeverry DM, Santodomingo AMS, Thomas RS, Gonzalez-Ugas J, Oyarzun-Ruiz P, Fuente MCS, et al. Trichinella spiralis in a cougar (Puma concolor) hunted by poachers in Chile. *Revista brasileira de parasitologia veterinaria = Brazilian Journal of Veterinary Parasitology: Orgao Oficial do Colegio Brasileiro de Parasitologia Veterinaria.* 2021;30(3):e002821.

28. Vieira-Pinto M, Fernandes ARG, Santos MH, Marucci G. *Trichinella britovi* infection in wild boar in Portugal. *Zoonoses and Public Health.* 2021;68(2):103–9.

29. Lesniak I, Franz M, Heckmann I, Greenwood AD, Hofer H, Krone O. Surrogate hosts: Hunting dogs and recolonizing grey wolves share their endoparasites. *International Journal for Parasitology: Parasites and Wildlife.* 2017;6(3):278–86.

30. Kilani T, El Hammami S. Pulmonary hydatid and other lung parasitic infections. *Current Opinion in Pulmonary Medicine.* 2002;8(3):218–23.

31. Norman FF, Chamorro S, Braojos F, Lopez-Miranda E, Chamorro J, Gonzalez I, et al. Strongyloides in bronchoalveolar lavage fluid: Practical implications in the COVID-19 era. *Journal of Travel Medicine.* 2022;29(1).

32. Morris A, Norris KA. Colonization by *Pneumocystis jirovecii* and its role in disease. *Clinical Microbiology Reviews.* 2012;25(2):297–317.

33. Dunaiski CM, Janssen L, Erzinger H, Pieper M, Damaschek S, Schildgen O, et al. Inter-specimen imbalance of mitochondrial gene copy numbers predicts clustering of *Pneumocystis jirovecii* isolates in distinct subgroups. *Journal of Fungi.* 2018;4(3).

34. Alanio A, Gits-Muselli M, Mercier-Delarue S, Dromer F, Bretagne S. Diversity of *Pneumocystis jirovecii* during infection revealed by ultra-deep pyrosequencing. *Frontiers in Microbiology.* 2016;7:733.

35. Matsumura Y, Ito Y, Iinuma Y, Yasuma K, Yamamoto M, Matsushima A, et al. Quantitative real-time PCR and the (1→3)-beta-D-glucan assay for differentiation between *Pneumocystis jirovecii* pneumonia and colonization. *Clinical Microbiology and Infection: The Official Publication of the European Society of Clinical Microbiology and Infectious Diseases.* 2012;18(6):591–7.

36. Zak P, Vejrazkova E, Zavrelova A, Pliskova L, Ryskova L, Hubacek P, et al. BAL fluid analysis in the identification of infectious agents in patients with hematological malignancies and pulmonary infiltrates. *Folia Microbiologica.* 2020;65(1):109–20.

37. Prickartz A, Lusebrink J, Khalfaoui S, Schildgen O, Schildgen V, Windisch W, et al. Low titer *Pneumocystis jirovecii* infections: More than just colonization? *Journal of Fungi.* 2016;2(2).

38. Liu J, Yu YT, Xu CH, Chen DC. Candida colonization in the respiratory tract: What is the significance? *Frontiers in Medicine.* 2020;7:598037.

39. King P. Haemophilus influenzae and the lung (Haemophilus and the lung). *Clinical and Translational Medicine.* 2012;1(1):10.

40. Stram MN, Suciu CN, Seheult JN, McCullough MA, Kader M, Wells A, et al. Herpes simplex Virus-1 qPCR in the diagnosis of lower respiratory tract infections in organ transplant recipients and critically ill patients. *American Journal of Clinical Pathology.* 2018;150(6):522–32.

41. van den Brink JW, Simoons-Smit AM, Beishuizen A, Girbes AR, Strack van Schijndel RJ, Groeneveld AB. Respiratory herpes simplex virus type 1 infection/colonisation in the critically ill: Marker or mediator? *Journal of Clinical Virology: The Official Publication of the Pan American Society for Clinical Virology.* 2004;30(1):68–72.

42. Costa C, Sidoti F, Saldan A, Sinesi F, Balloco C, Simeone S, et al. Clinical impact of HSV-1 detection in the lower respiratory tract from hospitalized adult patients. *Clinical Microbiology and Infection: The Official Publication of the European Society of Clinical Microbiology and Infectious Diseases.* 2012;18(8):E305–7.

43. Ghandili S, von Kroge PH, Simon M, Henes FO, Rohde H, Hoffmann A, et al. Diagnostic utility of bronchoalveolar lavage in patients with acute leukemia under broad-spectrum anti-infective treatment. *Cancers.* 2022;14(11).

44. Boeckh M, Stevens-Ayers T, Travi G, Huang ML, Cheng GS, Xie H, et al. Cytomegalovirus (CMV) DNA quantitation in bronchoalveolar lavage fluid from hematopoietic stem cell transplant recipients with CMV pneumonia. *The Journal of Infectious Diseases.* 2017;215(10):1514–22.

45. Pinana JL, Gimenez E, Gomez MD, Perez A, Gonzalez EM, Vinuesa V, et al. Pulmonary cytomegalovirus (CMV) DNA shedding in allogeneic hematopoietic stem cell transplant recipients: Implications for the diagnosis of CMV pneumonia. *The Journal of Infection.* 2019;78(5):393–401.

46. Inamdar DP, Anuradha B, Inamdar P, Patti PS. Microbiota of bronchoalveolar lavage samples from patients of lower respiratory tract infection – A changing trend. *Journal of Pure and Applied Microbiology.* 2021;15(3):1508–16.

47. Miller PR, Meredith JW, Chang MC. Optimal threshold for diagnosis of ventilator-associated pneumonia using bronchoalveolar lavage. *The Journal of Trauma.* 2003;55(2):263–7; discussion 7–8.

48. Meyer KC, Raghu G, Baughman RP, Brown KK, Costabel U, du Bois RM, et al. An official American Thoracic Society clinical practice guideline: The clinical utility of bronchoalveolar lavage cellular analysis in interstitial lung disease. *American Journal of Respiratory and Critical Care Medicine.* 2012;185(9):1004–14.

49. Costabel U. *Atlas Der Bronchoalveolären Lavage.* Stuttgart, New York: Thieme; 1994. 99 p.

50. Gallucci M, Pedretti M, Giannetti A, di Palmo E, Bertelli L, Pession A, et al. When the cough does not improve: A review on protracted bacterial bronchitis in children. *Frontiers in Pediatrics.* 2020;8:433.

51. Spagnolo P, Molyneaux PL, Bernardinello N, Cocconcelli E, Biondini D, Fracasso F, et al. The role of the lung's microbiome in the pathogenesis and progression of idiopathic pulmonary fibrosis. *International Journal of Molecular Sciences.* 2019;20(22).

52. Windisch W, Pieper M, Ziemele I, Rockstroh J, Brockmann M, Schildgen O, et al. Latent infection of human bocavirus accompanied by flare of chronic cough, fatigue and episodes of viral replication in an immunocompetent adult patient, Cologne, Germany. *JMM Case Reports.* 2016;3(4):e005052.

53. Vedder V, Schildgen V, Lusebrink J, Tillmann RL, Domscheit B, Windisch W, et al. Differential cytology profiles in bronchoalveolar lavage (BAL) in COVID-19 patients: A descriptive observation and comparison with other corona viruses, influenza virus, *Haemophilus influenzae*, and *Pneumocystis jirovecii. Medicine.* 2021;100(1):e24256.

54. Chen XM, Sun L, Yang K, Chen JM, Zhang L, Han XY, et al. Cytopathological analysis of bronchoalveolar lavage fluid in patients with and without HIV infection. *BMC Pulmonary Medicine*. 2022;22(1):55.

55. Wang H, Gu J, Li X, van der Gaast-de Jongh CE, Wang W, He X, et al. Broad range detection of viral and bacterial pathogens in bronchoalveolar lavage fluid of children to identify the cause of lower respiratory tract infections. *BMC Infectious Diseases*. 2021;21(1):152.

56. Singh G, Wulansari SG. Pattern of bacterial and fungal pathogen in patients with high risk for invasive fungal disease in an Indonesian tertiary care hospital: An observational study. *The Pan African Medical Journal*. 2018;29:60.

57. Gangell C, Gard S, Douglas T, Park J, de Klerk N, Keil T, et al. Inflammatory responses to individual microorganisms in the lungs of children with cystic fibrosis. *Clinical Infectious Diseases: An Official Publication of the Infectious Diseases Society of America*. 2011;53(5):425–32.

58. Sumino KC, Walter MJ, Mikols CL, Thompson SA, Gaudreault-Keener M, Arens MQ, et al. Detection of respiratory viruses and the associated chemokine responses in serious acute respiratory illness. *Thorax*. 2010;65(7):639–44.

59. Jouneau S, Poineuf JS, Minjolle S, Tattevin P, Uhel F, Kerjouan M, et al. Which patients should be tested for viruses on bronchoalveolar lavage fluid? *European Journal of Clinical Microbiology and Infectious Diseases: Official Publication of the European Society of Clinical Microbiology*. 2013;32(5):671–7.

60. Garbino J, Soccal PM, Aubert JD, Rochat T, Meylan P, Thomas Y, et al. Respiratory viruses in bronchoalveolar lavage: A hospital-based cohort study in adults. *Thorax*. 2009;64(5):399–404.

61. Bouzid D, Hingrat QL, Salipante F, Ferre VM, Chevallier T, Tubiana S, et al. Agreement of respiratory viruses' detection between nasopharyngeal swab and bronchoalveolar lavage in adults admitted for pneumonia: A retrospective study. *Clinical Microbiology and Infection: The Official Publication of the European Society of Clinical Microbiology and Infectious Diseases*. 2023, 29(7):941e1–e6.

62. Kumar T, Prasad T, Nigam JS, Sinha R, Bhadani PP. Parasitic larvae in bronchoalveolar lavage fluid in a non-immunocompromised patient. *Cytopathology: Official Journal of the British Society for Clinical Cytology*. 2023;34(2):173–5.

63. Meehan AM, Virk A, Swanson K, Poeschla EM. Severe pleuropulmonary paragonimiasis 8 years after emigration from a region of endemicity. *Clinical Infectious Diseases: An Official Publication of the Infectious Diseases Society of America*. 2002;35(1):87–90.

64. Failoc-Rojas VE, Iglesias-Osores S, Silva-Diaz H. *Lophomonas* spp. in the upper and lower respiratory tract of patients from a hospital in Lambayeque, Peru: Clinical case studies. *Respiratory Medicine Case Reports*. 2020;31:101142.

65. Lin C, Ying F, Lai Y, Li X, Xue X, Zhou T, et al. Use of nested PCR for the detection of trichomonads in bronchoalveolar lavage fluid. *BMC Infectious Diseases*. 2019;19(1):512.

66. Abdulla MA, Hombal SM, al-Juwaiser A. Detection of *Schistosoma mansoni* in bronchoalveolar lavage fluid: A case report. *Acta Cytologica*. 1999;43(5):856–8.

67. Jacobs F, Depierreux M, Goldman M, Hall M, Liesnard C, Janssen F, et al. Role of bronchoalveolar lavage in diagnosis of disseminated toxoplasmosis. *Reviews of Infectious Diseases*. 1991;13(4):637–41.

6

BAL findings in interstitial lung disease

LUTZ-BERNHARD JEHN, FRANCESCO BONELLA, MICHAEL KREUTER,
JOSUNE GUZMAN, AND ULRICH COSTABEL

INTRODUCTION

Classification of interstitial lung diseases

Interstitial lung diseases (ILDs) are a heterogeneous group of diseases characterized by inflammation and/or fibrosis that can affect the lung interstitium, the alveoli, and the bronchi and bronchioli. Patients with ILD typically present with the clinical symptoms of progressive dyspnea, restrictive ventilatory impairment, and chronic respiratory insufficiency. Based on clinical, radiological, and histopathological criteria more than 180 distinct ILD entities have been described, which can be categorized into four groups (1, 2). Figure 6.1 provides an overview of these categories with the corresponding ILD subtypes.

The first group of ILDs includes diseases associated with known causes like drug-induced ILDs, pulmonary involvement of connective tissue diseases (CTDs), and the heterogeneous group of pneumoconioses. Importantly, virtually any systemic disease can be associated with an ILD, and drug-induced lung injury should be always considered as a possible cause in the evaluation of patients with suspected ILD.

The second group of ILDs refers to idiopathic interstitial pneumonias (IIPs). IIPs can be further subdivided into the subgroup of fibrosing ILDs comprising idiopathic pulmonary fibrosis (IPF) and idiopathic non-specific interstitial pneumonia (NSIP). Also smoking-related ILDs (respiratory bronchiolitis with interstitial lung disease (RB-ILD), desquamative interstitial pneumonia (DIP)), ILDs associated with acute or subacute clinical onset (acute interstitial pneumonitis (AIP), cryptogenic organizing pneumonia (COP)), and rare entities (lymphocytic interstitial pneumonitis (LIP), pleuroparenchymal fibroelastosis (PPFE)) belong to the group of IIPs. In up to 15% of ILD cases, it is not possible to categorize an IIP into one of these four groups despite extensive clinical, radiological, and/or pathological assessment. These entities are labeled as unclassifiable ILD (3).

The third group of ILDs consists of granulomatous ILDs, including pulmonary sarcoidosis, hypersensitivity pneumonitis (HP), and chronic beryllium disease (CBD).

DOI: 10.1201/9781003146834-8

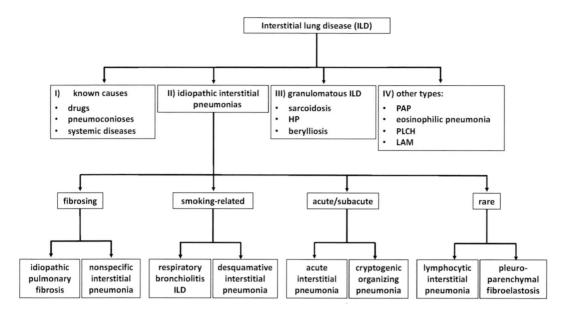

Figure 6.1 The classification of interstitial lung disease (ILD) into four groups according to the current international multidisciplinary classification of idiopathic interstitial pneumonias is shown (2). Abbreviations: HP, hypersensitivity pneumonitis; ILD, interstitial lung disease; LAM, lymphangioleiomyomatosis; PAP, pulmonary alveolar proteinosis; PLHC, pulmonary Langerhans cell histiocytosis.

Finally, rare entities account for the fourth group of ILDs. For example, pulmonary alveolar proteinosis (PAP), acute or chronic eosinophilic pneumonia, pulmonary Langerhans cell histiocytosis (PLCH), and lymphangioleiomyomatosis (LAM) are subsumed under this ILD group.

Epidemiology and prognostic considerations for ILD

Data on the global burden and geographic heterogeneity of ILD are limited.

The most frequent ILD is IPF with a prevalence between 20–80 per 100,000 in North America and Europe, followed by sarcoidosis (4–6).

Conversely, HP is more common in Asia than in North America or Europe, with a relative frequency of 47.3% of all ILD cases included in a prospective multicenter registry study, which recruited 1,084 ILD patients from 27 centers between 2012 and 2015 for the epidemiological evaluation of ILD frequencies in India (7).

The male-to-female ratio is variable across ILD subtypes, with pneumoconioses and IPF being more prevalent among men compared to women in North America and Europe (male-to-female ratio of 2.3 and 1.4, respectively) (8).

The prognosis of ILDs is highly variable across entities. In patients with untreated IPF, the median overall survival time is three to five years (9), whereas in patients with HP prognosis depends on identification of inciting antigen (10) and in sarcoidosis on organ manifestation and onset of complications (11).

AIM OF THE CHAPTER

The aim of this chapter is to provide an overview on the role of bronchoalveolar lavage fluid (BALF) analysis in the diagnostic evaluation of patients with suspected ILD. We first discuss the value of BALF differential cytology and other BALF cellular findings for selected ILD entities. We then address the utility of BALF cellular analysis for specific clinical scenarios, which can occur in the management of patients with ILD. Finally, we briefly outline the role of BALF cellular analysis as a tool for monitoring disease activity, guiding therapy, or providing prognostic information for certain ILD subtypes.

THE ROLE OF BAL IN THE DIAGNOSTIC EVALUATION OF PATIENTS WITH ILD

Indications and safety of performing BAL in ILD

BAL is a safe and well-tolerated procedure performed during flexible bronchoscopy under conscious sedation. BAL is principally indicated in all patients with suspected ILD or unclear pulmonary opacities on chest radiography. If clinical and lung functional findings point towards a diagnosis of ILD, BAL might even be indicated in patients with normal radiographic findings (12).

Bronchoscopy with BAL has been reported as the potential cause of acute exacerbations in patients with IPF (13–15). However, the safety of BAL in such patients was recently clarified based on data from the Prospective Observation of Fibrosis in Lung Clinical Endpoints (PROFILE) study cohort (16). In this study, 223 IPF patients underwent bronchoscopy and all subjects in the bronchoscopy cohort tolerated the procedure well, a cell differential was available for all, and there were no immediate (<72 h) complications (17). Based on these observations, safety can be considered as one major advantage of BAL in comparison to more invasive approaches in the diagnostic algorithm for ILDs considering different transbronchial biopsy (TBB) techniques, and surgical lung biopsy (SLB) (18, 19).

Although there are virtually no absolute contraindications for performing BAL during flexible bronchoscopy, caution is warranted when BAL is performed in the evaluation of patients with suspected ILD and respiratory failure (PaO$_2$ < 60 mmHg at room air), pulmonary comorbidities including severe asthma, chronic obstructive pulmonary disease, and emphysema (FEV1 < 60% of predicted normal value or 1 L absolute), or increased risk of bleeding (decreased platelet count, deranged prothrombin time, elevated International Normalized Ratio and elevated activated partial thromboplastin time, respectively) (20). Nevertheless, BAL can even be performed in patients on therapeutic anticoagulation, preferably via oral route to avoid epistaxis, and in critically ill patients requiring high-flow nasal oxygen,

non-invasive ventilation, or invasive mechanical ventilation after careful risk-benefit analysis (21).

Handling, processing, and technique of BAL cell analyses in ILD

A detailed description of the BAL procedure regarding the handling, processing, and technique of BALF cellular analysis can be found in the first part of this book.

In brief, in a patient with suspected ILD, BAL should be performed in the involved lung segments, guided by a chest high-resolution computed tomography (HRCT) performed before the procedure, or in the right middle or left lingular lobe, in the case of diffuse bilateral infiltrates.

According to the official American Thoracic Society (ATS) clinical practice guideline for BALF cellular analysis in ILD, a total volume of 100–300 ml should be instilled into the identified target lung segment via a flexible video bronchoscope with immediate aspiration by gentle suction after each aliquot. Cellular analysis should be performed within 1 hour if the BALF is in nutrient-poor media (e.g., saline). The total count of nucleated cells is usually obtained via a hemocytometer, and cell viability can be determined by Trypan blue exclusion. Differential cell counts are performed via cytocentrifugation, staining with Wright–Giemsa or May–Grünwald–Giemsa (MGG), and counting of at least 400 cells (12).

The diagnostic value of BALF differential cytology findings in ILD

The usefulness of BALF differential cytology findings in the diagnostic work-up of ILD was emphasized in the ATS/ERS international consensus classification of IIPs of 2002 (1) and has been substantiated in the updated ATS/ERS international consensus classification of IIPs, published in 2013 (2).

Figure 6.2 shows the algorithm for the clinical utility of BALF cellular analysis in the evaluation of ILD modified according to the official ATS clinical practice guideline for BALF cellular analysis in ILD (12). BAL and TBB techniques are frequently combined and can reveal complementary results.

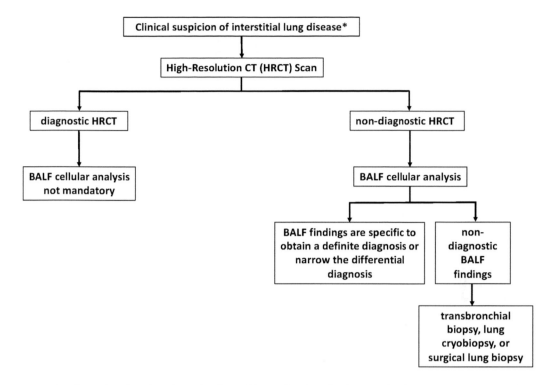

Figure 6.2 Algorithm for the clinical utility of bronchoalveolar lavage fluid (BALF) cellular analysis in the evaluation of interstitial lung disease (ILD) modified from the current ATS clinical practice guideline for the clinical utility of BALF cellular analysis in ILD (12). *Clinical evidence of ILD is based on patient history, physical examination, chest radiograph, and lung function test results. Abbreviations: HRCT, high-resolution computed tomography; BALF, bronchoalveolar lavage fluid.

One limitation of BALF differential cytology in the diagnostic evaluation of ILDs is its lack of specificity. However, when BALF differential cytology findings are interpreted in the context of clinical and HRCT findings, and in an experienced multidisciplinary discussion (MDD) setting, it may contribute to narrowing the differential diagnosis of ILD and help to avoid TBBs or SLB (22–24).

It is noteworthy that there are ILD subtypes in which the presence of specific HRCT patterns, combined with typical clinical constellations, might be sufficient enough that neither tissue sampling nor BALF cellular analysis is necessary (25).

If BAL is indicated, a differential cell count should be routinely obtained in all patients with suspected ILD (26). There are no internationally standardized reference values for BALF differential cytology findings (27), yet a couple of

guidelines and recommendations may facilitate the interpretation of BALF findings in the diagnostic work-up of patients with suspected ILD (12, 28–31).

Beyond determining the absolute count of nucleated BALF immune cells, BALF differential cytology findings can be categorized into distinct immune cell patterns (12). A BALF differential cell count with greater than 15% lymphocytes, greater than 3% neutrophils, greater than 1% eosinophils, or greater than 0.5% mast cells, is classified as BALF lymphocytosis (i.e., a lymphocytic cellular pattern), BALF neutrophilia (i.e., a neutrophilic cellular pattern), BALF eosinophilia (i.e., an eosinophilic cellular pattern), or BALF mastocytosis, respectively. An increase in more than one type of cell in the BAL represents a mixed cellular pattern. Representative photomicrographs of these BALF immune cell patterns are shown in Figure 6.3.

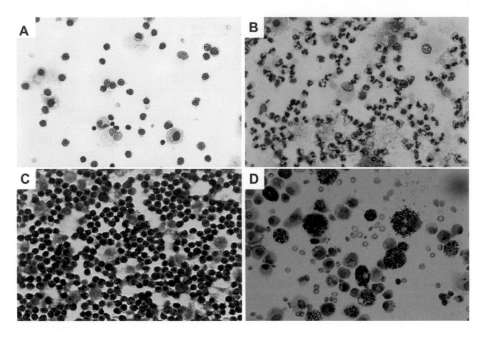

Figure 6.3 Photomicrographs of representative bronchoalveolar lavage fluid (BALF) smear preparations stained with May–Grünwald–Giemsa are shown (400× original magnification). (A) BALF lymphocytosis. (B) BALF neutrophil predominance. (C) BALF eosinophilia. (D) BALF sample with a marked increase of mast cells.

It is important to note at this point, that the diagnostic value of classifying BALF differential cell counts into immune cell patterns based on the thresholds mentioned above is limited by their lack of specificity. Several disease-specific cut-off values have been proposed to overcome this limitation.

In the case of a predominant lymphocytic pattern, a lymphocyte differential count ≥25–30% suggests granulomatous lung disease (e.g., sarcoidosis, HP, NSIP, CBD, drug reaction, LIP, COP, or lymphoma), whereas a marked lymphocytosis >50% is particularly suggestive of HP or cellular NSIP. An eosinophil differential count of ≥25% is virtually diagnostic of eosinophilic lung disease when it occurs in the context of a typical clinical constellation, whereas an eosinophilic pattern with an eosinophil cell count below that threshold of 25% is unspecific and can be present in various ILDs including fibrotic IIPs or DIP. A neutrophil differential cell count of ≥50% strongly supports acute lung injury, aspiration pneumonia, or suppurative infection. A mast cell differential count of >1% combined with a lymphocyte differential

count of >50% and a neutrophil count of >3% can be regarded as highly suggestive of HP. The presence of >5% epithelial cells (either squamous epithelial cells from the upper airway tract or bronchial epithelial cells from the lower airway tract) in the sample suggests a suboptimal BAL quality. BAL may not have adequately sampled distal airspaces in this situation, and BALF cellular findings can be regarded as not representative of the alveolar space (Figure 6.4). If reasonable, BAL should be repeated in these cases (12).

Table 6.1 provides an overview of selected ILD subtypes associated with either a lymphocytic, neutrophilic, eosinophilic, or mixed BALF immune cell pattern.

The finding that these immune cell patterns may support or suggest a certain type of ILD in the absence of an infection is the result of several studies investigating the impact of BALF differential cell counts on the final ILD diagnosis. For example, a pronounced BALF eosinophilia has been shown to be an important finding to obtain a diagnosis of eosinophilic pneumonia (32, 33), or drug reactions (34, 35), and the identification

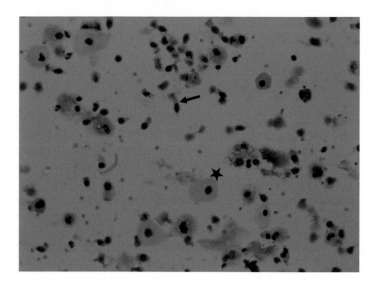

Figure 6.4 A bronchoalveolar lavage fluid (BALF) smear preparation stained with May–Grünwald–Giemsa as an example of an unsatisfactory BAL specimen with increased squamous epithelial cells (marked with a black star) and degenerating columnar epithelial cells with ciliated epithelium (marked with a black arrow) is shown (200× original magnification). Epithelial cells >5% are suggestive for suboptimal sample quality, BALF cellular patterns should be interpreted with caution in these cases.

Table 6.1 Bronchoalveolar lavage fluid (BALF) cellular pattern as an adjunct to interstitial lung disease (ILD) diagnosis

BALF cellular findings	Associated interstitial lung disease
Neutrophilic (± eosinophilic)	Idiopathic pulmonary fibrosis, fibrotic non-specific interstitial pneumonia, desquamative interstitial pneumonia, collagen vascular diseases, asbestosis, ARDS, bacterial pneumonia, bronchiolitis, drug-induced reaction
Eosinophilic	Acute and chronic eosinophilic pneumonia, eosinophilic granulomatosis with polyangiitis, desquamative interstitial pneumonia, drug-induced reaction
Lymphocytic	Sarcoidosis, hypersensitivity pneumonitis, cryptogenic organizing pneumonia, cellular non-specific interstitial pneumonia, drug-induced reaction, lymphoid interstitial pneumonia, collagen vascular diseases, silicosis
Mixed cellularity (lymphocytic / neutrophilic granulocytes / eosinophilic granulocytes)	Cryptogenic organizing pneumonia, chronic hypersensitivity pneumonitis, non-specific interstitial pneumonia, collagen vascular diseases
Macrophages containing smoking-related inclusions	Respiratory bronchiolitis with interstitial lung disease, desquamative interstitial pneumonia, Langerhans cell histiocytosis
Foamy macrophages	Amiodarone exposure, HP, COP

Source: The table is modified according to Costabel et al. (35).
ARDS, acute respiratory distress syndrome.

of BALF lymphocytosis has been associated with an increased likelihood for the diagnosis of sarcoidosis (36, 37), HP (38, 39), pneumotoxic drug reactions (40, 41), or cellular NSIP (42, 43). A mixed cellular pattern can be observed with any ILD subtype, and the dominant cell type may be the most consistent with a specific ILD diagnosis (44). However, several of these studies were conducted prior to the era of HRCT as a widespread diagnostic resource for ILD, and even before IIPs were recognized as distinct clinical entities, leading to an important risk of potential bias.

The diagnostic value of other BALF cellular analyses in ILD

A lymphocyte subset analysis (performed by either flow cytometry or immunocytochemistry) on the basis of T helper (CD4+) versus T suppressor (CD8+) phenotypes can be performed if a lymphocytic ILD is suspected or the initial BALF findings indicate a lymphocytosis. As shown in Table 6.2, ILDs can be categorized into subtypes with a normal, increased, or decreased CD4+/CD8+ T lymphocyte ratio (35).

However, classifying of ILDs into groups with a normal, increased, or decreased CD4+/CD8+ T lymphocyte ratio has limitations. For example, this ratio can be decreased in up to 15% of patients with sarcoidosis (45). Vice versa, in HP a substantial proportion of patients might reveal a normal or even increased CD4+/CD8+ T lymphocyte ratio, especially those with chronic HP (46). The BALF CD4+/CD8+ T lymphocyte ratio also varies with age and might even be increased in healthy subjects without evidence of underlying ILD, which should be considered as a further

limitation of this diagnostic test in the evaluation of suspected ILD (47).

Analyses of other immune cell subsets, for example staining of BALF immune cells with the Langerhans cell marker CD1a for suspected PLCH, can be ordered in specific settings (48).

BALF staining of different types of glycoproteins by periodic acid–Schiff (PAS) reaction is most valuable if PAP syndrome is suspected. The identification of PAS-positive non-cellular corpuscles and amorphous debris alongside with the characteristic opaque, milky BALF appearance is highly specific for the presence of PAP syndrome (49). PAS staining of BALF samples is not established in the diagnostic work-up of ILDs other than PAP.

Oil red O (ORO) staining of lipid-laden macrophages is performed by using *Sudan* dyes, such as *Sudan* III, *Sudan* IV, and *Sudan* black, and can be used to diagnose lipoid pneumonia and to assess patients with ILD for chronic aspiration, or patients who have undergone lung transplantation as a part of their postoperative surveillance (50). Gastroesophageal reflux might occur in many patients with IPF, and esophageal dysfunction can be particularly severe in patients with systemic sclerosis (SSc). However, although repetitive microaspiration, or even silent aspiration of gastric contents, might be involved in the pathogenesis of ILDs such as IPF or SSc-ILD, ORO staining of BALF samples is not recommended as a routine screening tool for aspiration in these patients (51). Limitations of ORO staining include variation in scoring systems (lipid-laden macrophage index vs percentage of ORO-positive alveolar macrophages), variation in scoring results between observers, staining

Table 6.2 CD4+/CD8+ ratio in diseases with lymphocytic alveolitis

CD4/CD8 increased	CD4/CD8 normal	CD4/CD8 decreased
Sarcoidosis	Tuberculosis	Hypersensitivity pneumonitis
Chronic beryllium disease	Lymphangitic carcinomatosis	Drug-induced pneumonitis
Asbestos-induced alveolitis		Cryptogenic organizing pneumonia
Crohn's disease		HIV infection
Connective tissue disorders		Silicosis

Source: The table is modified according to Costabel et al. (35).
HIV, human immunodeficiency virus.

quality, air-bubble formation, and the presence of hemosiderin and anthracotic pigment in alveolar macrophages (52). Lipid-laden macrophages have been also found in healthy controls as well as in respiratory disorders unlikely to be associated with aspiration, and ORO staining of BALF samples cannot distinguish aspiration of exogenous lipids from lipids of gastric origin (53).

The use of Prussian blue staining of BALF samples to detect hemosiderin-laden macrophages is indicated if diffuse alveolar hemorrhage (DAH) syndrome is suspected. Although frequently associated with anti-neutrophil cytoplasmic antibodies (ANCA)-associated vasculitis, DAH is a syndrome that can be caused by a variety of associated conditions which lead to a disruption of the alveolar capillary basement membrane integrity (54). Several diagnostic criteria incorporating different BALF cut-off values for hemosiderin-laden macrophages have been proposed to identify DAH syndrome, though the presence of ≥20% hemosiderin-laden macrophages is generally considered as diagnostic for DAH in the absence of ongoing active bleeding (55).

Figure 6.5 shows representative photomicrographs of lipid-laden macrophages detected in the BALF of a patient with suspected aspiration, hemosiderin-laden macrophages visualized in the BALF of a patient with suspected

ANCA-associated vasculitis (AAV)-ILD, and an example for a positive PAS reaction in a patient with suspected PAP syndrome.

Because infections and diffuse neoplasms including primary pulmonary lymphoma, lymphangitic carcinomatosis, and bronchoalveolar carcinoma can mimic ILD or complicate preexisting ILD, BALF staining and culture for bacteria, mycobacteria, and fungi in the microbiology laboratory, as well as screening for neoplastic cells, might be indicated in the appropriate clinical setting.

Highly specific and pathognomonic BALF findings in ILD

In certain mostly rare ILD entities, BALF findings may be highly specific or even pathognomonic (Table 6.3). Many of these disorders are included in the group of alveolar-filling syndromes. Abnormal material that accumulates in the alveolar spaces can be washed out easily by lavage and can provide diagnostic findings (24). Such BALF findings can be found in acute eosinophilic pneumonia (56–58), chronic eosinophilic pneumonia (59, 60), other eosinophilic lung disorders, neoplasms (61), PAP syndrome (62), lipoid pneumonia (63, 64), PLCH (48, 65, 66), and DAH syndrome (67, 68). It should be considered at this

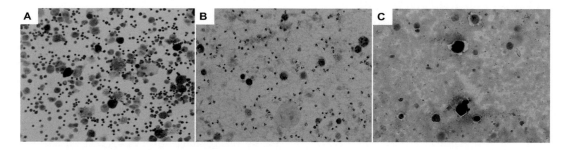

Figure 6.5 (A) O (ORO) staining of a bronchoalveolar lavage fluid (BALF) specimen obtained from a patient with suspected aspiration. The red appearance of lipid-laden macrophages can be seen when visualized under light microscopy (200× original magnification). (B) Prussian blue staining of a BALF specimen obtained from a patient with suspected ILD associated with granulomatosis with polyangiitis (GPA). Hemosiderin-laden macrophages, suggestive of diffuse alveolar hemorrhage (DAH) syndrome, can be seen accompanied by a predominant neutrophilic immune cell pattern (200× original magnification). (C) Periodic acid–Schiff (PAS) staining of a BALF sample obtained from a patient with suspected pulmonary alveolar proteinosis (PAP). PAS-positive, amorphous, predominantly acellular debris can be seen, which is highly specific for the presence of PAP syndrome (200× original magnification).

Table 6.3 Diagnostic bronchoalveolar lavage fluid (BALF) findings in the evaluation of suspected interstitial lung disease (ILD)

BALF finding	Diagnosis
Pneumocystis jirovecii, fungi, CMV-transformed cells	Opportunistic infections
Milky effluent, PAS-positive non-cellular corpuscles, amorphous debris, foamy macrophages	Alveolar proteinosis
Hemosiderin-laden macrophages, intracytoplasmic fragments of red blood cells in macrophages, free red blood cells	Alveolar hemorrhage syndrome
Malignant cells of solid tumors, lymphoma, leukemia	Malignant infiltrates
Dust particles in macrophages, asbestos bodies	Dust / asbestos exposure
"Oily" lipid vacuoles in macrophages	Lipoid pneumonia
Eosinophils >25%	Eosinophilic lung disease
Positive beryllium lymphocyte proliferation test	Chronic beryllium disease
CD1a-positive Langerhans cells increased ≥5% of BALF immune cells	Langerhans cell histiocytosis
Hyperplastic pneumocytes	Diffuse alveolar damage, drug toxicity

Source: The table is modified according to Costabel et al. (35).
BAL, bronchoalveolar lavage; CMV, cytomegalovirus; PAS, Periodic acid–Schiff.

point, that some of these disorders like PAP and DAH are heterogenous syndromes. Even though each of these syndromes might be characterized by common pulmonary manifestations, BALF analysis as a standalone test is not sufficient to identify any of the underlying causative disorders.

BALF CELLULAR FINDINGS ASSOCIATED WITH SELECTED ILD ENTITIES

The diagnostic utility of BAL in ILD associated with known causes (group I)

DRUG-INDUCED ILD

As reviewed by Costabel et al. (35), many drugs can induce a toxic or immune-mediated interstitial lung reaction. In addition to toxic changes of the type II pneumocytes, the most frequent BALF differential cytology finding is a lymphocytic alveolitis with the predominance of CD8+ T cells, similar to HP. However, in drug-induced ILD any type of cellular pattern (lymphocytic,

neutrophilic, eosinophilic, or mixed) and DAH may be present.

In patients treated with amiodarone, an antiarrhythmic medication established in the management of several types of cardiac dysrhythmias, characteristic alterations in the alveolar macrophage population can be observed (69). Amiodarone induces an increase in the phospholipid content in nearly all body cells, with the highest concentrations observed in phagocytic cells. This finding is reflected by the presence of foamy macrophages in the BALF of patients exposed to amiodarone, even in the absence of clinical lung involvement (Figure 6.6). Although a normal BAL differential does not exclude amiodarone-induced lung disease, the absence of foamy macrophages argues against an amiodarone-induced pneumonitis (70–72).

Because BALF findings are not specific to any drug-induced lung disease, the definitive diagnosis needs additional clinical investigations. BAL can be useful, however, to exclude other pulmonary problems that are commonly associated with the use of certain types of drugs like infections in patients treated with immunosuppressants (73).

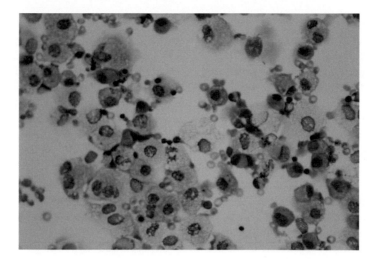

Figure 6.6 An example of foamy macrophages in a patient with exposure to amiodarone and suspected amiodarone-induced lung disease is shown. If foamy macrophages are not present in BAL, an amiodarone-induced pneumonitis likely can be excluded (May–Grünwald–Giemsa staining, 400× original magnification).

Table 6.4 provides an overview on BALF findings in drug-induced ILD.

RADIATION-INDUCED LUNG INJURY

The term radiation-induced lung injury (RILI) is used for any lung toxicity induced by radiation therapy. RILI can either present acutely as radiation pneumonitis or chronically as radiation pulmonary fibrosis (74).

An increase in several BALF immune cell types can be observed, but a lymphocytosis both in irradiated and non-irradiated, contralateral lung, seems to be the most common BALF immune cell pattern (75, 76).

Table 6.4 Overview of bronchoalveolar lavage fluid (BALF) differential cytology findings in drug-induced interstitial lung disease

Lymphocytosis	Neutrophilia	Eosinophilia	Hemorrhage	Cytotoxic reaction
Methotrexate	Bleomycin	Bleomycin	D-penicillamine	Bleomycin
Azathioprine	Busulfan	Nitrofurantoin	Amphotericin	Methotrexate
Cyclophosphamide	Minocycline	Cotrimazole	B Cytotoxic	Nitrosureas Busulfan
Bleomycin	Amiodarone	Penicillin	drugs	Cyclophosphamide
Busulfan Vincristine		Sulfasalazine		
Nitrofurantoin		Ampicillin		
Minocycline		Tetracycline		
Gold		Maloprim		
Sulfasalazine		Minocycline		
Amiodarone		L-tryptophan		
Acebutolol				
Atenolol				
Celiprolol Propanolol				
Flecainide				
Diphenylhydantoin				
Nilutamide				

Source: Data are extracted from Costabel et al. (35).

PNEUMOCONIOSES

Pneumoconioses are a heterogenous group of lung diseases caused by the inhalation of organic or non-organic airborne dust and fibers, which can cause inflammation and fibrosis in the lung.

Asbestosis, silicosis, and coal miner's lung are the most common types of pneumoconiosis and are well-known causes of dust-induced ILDs.

Even though most types of pneumoconiosis are completely preventable, a global increase in the prevalence of asbestosis has been observed, and cases of severe, progressive forms of silicosis recently observed in countries including Israel, Spain, and Australia were attributable to the processing of high silica-containing artificial stone material used to fabricate domestic benchtops (77, 78).

In asbestosis, BALF cellular findings are nonspecific and an increased absolute BALF cell count with overall increased macrophages and any type of BALF immune cell pattern has been described. In subjects with a high asbestos burden of the lung, MGG-stained smears may reveal asbestos bodies either with a rod-like appearance or shaped as elongated dumbbell-shaped crystals. Asbestos bodies are positive on iron staining. It is important to note that the presence of asbestos bodies in BALF samples demonstrates exposure to asbestos but is not sufficient for a definitive diagnosis of asbestosis. For specific questions, the number of asbestos bodies in the BALF can be counted and quantified as asbestos bodies per ml BALF using a millipore filtration method (79–82).

In chronic silicosis, abundant macrophages with an increase in lymphocytes and neutrophils can be seen. Birefringent particles consistent with silica may be seen with polarized microscopy. In acute silicosis, lavage often appears milky, and, similar to alveolar proteinosis, foamy macrophages with positive PAS staining can be present (83–85).

In coal miner's lung, increased cellularity with anthracotic-pigmented macrophages is the main BALF differential cytology finding. A neutrophilic cellular pattern (usually mild to moderate) may be seen, especially in those with progressive massive fibrosis (86, 87).

BALF FINDINGS IN ILD ASSOCIATED WITH CTDS

ILD can arise in a variety of CTDs (CTD-ILD), either primarily or secondarily due to infections, drug toxicity, and lymphoproliferative or neoplastic disorders, that are more common in patients with CTD than in the immunocompetent population. The prevalence of ILD in patients with CTD is around 15% and varies according to the underlying CTD, as shown in Table 6.5. ILD has been associated with worse outcomes in patients with CTD, highlighting the need for a precise ILD diagnosis and adequate treatment in these patients (88, 89).

As reviewed by Tomassetti et al. (90), the perceived value of performing BAL in the characterization of CTD-ILD is low and several nonspecific BALF immune cell patterns have been described. Lymphocytosis was more frequently observed in CTD-ILD cases with acute and subacute onset, correlating with cellular NSIP and OP radiological patterns, and lymphocytosis has even been described in cases without clinical/radiographic lung involvement (91).

In other ILD diagnoses such as chronic HP or idiopathic NSIP, a marked BALF lymphocytosis has been shown to correlate with a greater likelihood of response to immunosuppressive therapy and favorable outcomes (92, 93). In CTD-ILD, the

Table 6.5 Prevalence of interstitial lung involvement in connective tissue diseases and anti-neutrophil cytoplasmic antibodies (ANCA)-associated vasculitis

Connective tissue disease	Prevalence
Systemic sclerosis	up to 85%
Rheumatoid arthritis	20–30%
Idiopathic inflammatory myopathy	20–50%
Sjogren's syndrome	up to 25%
Systemic lupus erythematosus	2–8%
Anti-myeloperoxidase antibody-positive microscopic polyangiitis	up to 45%

Source: The table is modified according to Tomassetti et al. (90).

ANCA, anti-neutrophil cytoplasmic antibodies.

value of BALF analysis to evaluate disease activity, to assess treatment responses, or to predict the risk of disease progression still needs further investigation. At least, in the routine management of patients with CTD-ILD BALF analysis is useful to rule out complications, mainly infections and drug-induced ILD (90).

Systemic sclerosis (SSc)

ILD can be observed in nearly 50% of patients with systemic sclerosis (SSc-ILD), and, together with pulmonary hypertension, now represents the main cause of death in patients with SSc (94). ILD can develop in any patient with SSc, and NSIP is the most common HRCT pattern associated with SSc-ILD (95). Risk factors for ILD development in SSc are diffuse (rather than limited) cutaneous SSc, the presence of anti-Scl-70/anti-topoisomerase I antibody, and the absence of anti-centromere antibody (96). BALF differential cytology findings in SSc-ILD are non-specific and include an increased percentage of neutrophils, eosinophils, and/or lymphocytes (97). Even though BALF neutrophilia has been linked to early mortality, the additional value of BAL in predicting disease progression or long-term survival in SSc-ILD compared with HRCT and pulmonary function tests is controversial (98). Thus, BALF neutrophilia in SSc-ILD seems to be rather a marker of disease severity, than to provide independent prognostic information (99).

Rheumatoid arthritis (RA)

ILD can be observed in up to 30% of patients with rheumatoid arthritis (RA-ILD) (100), and also in patients with RA, the presence of ILD was shown to be an independent adverse risk factor for survival (101). In a study of patients with RA-ILD, four major HRCT patterns of disease were identified, namely usual interstitial pneumonia (UIP) (37%), NSIP (30%), obliterative bronchiolitis (17%), and OP (8%) (102). Neutrophilia, the most common BALF immune cell pattern in patients with RA-ILD, has been shown to correlate with disease severity and is most pronounced in patients with an underlying UIP HRCT pattern, while obliterative bronchiolitis has been associated with a mixed immune cell pattern characterized by an increase in both, BALF neutrophil and lymphocyte levels (103). Lymphocytosis and eosinophilia

may also be present in RA-ILD, but no correlation with the presence of ILD or pulmonary function impairment has been described (104).

Idiopathic inflammatory myopathies (IIM)

ILD associated with idiopathic inflammatory myopathies (IIM) represents a large group of CTD-ILD, that can have an acute onset of symptoms and that can be limited to the lungs (amyopathic variants). A mixed type of NSIP and OP represents the predominant HRCT pattern, followed less frequently by NSIP, OP, UIP, and diffuse alveolar damage (DAD) patterns. Neutrophilia or lymphocytosis with a predominance of $CD8^+$ T cells is the most common BALF finding, whereas eosinophilia has also been reported (105). BAL may be further helpful in excluding malignancies, infections, and aspiration, which all are well-known complications of patients with IIM-associated ILD. In particular, anti-synthetase (AS) syndrome and anti-MDA-5 antibody (aMDA-5) dermato-pulmonary syndrome are responsible for cases of acute deteriorating ILD associated with IIM. No impact of BALF differential cytology findings on hospital mortality was observed in a French multicenter retrospective study investigating outcomes and clinical features of patients with acute respiratory failure (ARF) revealing AS syndrome or aMDA-5 dermato-pulmonary syndrome. This study failed to identify any predictive role of BALF differential cytology findings on hospital survival and there was no correlation between BALF findings and HRCT patterns, even though BALF neutrophil counts were significantly increased in the group of patients diagnosed with AS syndrome compared to the group of patients revealing aMDA-5 dermato-pulmonary syndrome (106).

Systemic lupus erythematosus (SLE)

Whereas pleural effusion can complicate the clinical course in SLE in up to 30% of cases, the prevalence of ILD (2–8%) is comparably rare. The role of BAL in SLE is particularly relevant in the assessment of DAH syndrome, which can be diagnosed based on the criteria introduced in the section "The diagnostic value of other BALF cellular analyses in ILD," and acute lupus pneumonitis that occurs in 1–4% of patients (107). Both are life-threatening conditions that should be promptly identified and differentiated from infections and aspiration pneumonia that in SLE are also significantly increased.

Sjögren's syndrome (SS)

In Sjögren's syndrome (SS) ILD has been observed in up to 25% of cases. The most common HRCT patterns are in order of decreasing frequency NSIP, UIP, LIP, and OP, respectively. BAL usually reveals a lymphocytosis with increased prevalence of CD8+ T cells, whereas neutrophilia is uncommon (108). In SS-associated ILD, lymphocytosis is usually associated with follicular bronchiolitis and LIP, cellular NSIP, or OP. However, exclusion of lymphoma should be performed in cases of SS-associated ILD revealing high BALF lymphocyte levels, given the high prevalence of lymphomas in SS (109).

ANCA-ASSOCIATED ILD

The vast majority of ILD cases associated with ANCA-positivity or AAV has been shown to be in the setting of anti-myeloperoxidase antibody-positive disease and can be present in up to 45% of patients of microscopic polyangiitis, though cases of ILD associated with proteinase 3 ANCA have rarely been reported. BALF findings in patients with AAV-ILD are non-specific, though data are limited. An increased cellular count with elevated neutrophils has been reported in most available studies evaluating BAL findings in AAV-ILD (110). In eosinophilic granulomatosis with polyangiitis (EGPA, formerly Churg–Strauss syndrome) an increased fraction of eosinophils is common (111). Neutrophil predominance with slight elevation in lymphocytes or eosinophils is seen in the BALF of patients with granulomatosis with polyangiitis (GPA), formerly known as Wegener's granulomatosis (112, 113). Because AAV can lead to a disruption of the alveolar capillary basement membrane, DAH might be present in any case of AAV-ILD (114).

The diagnostic utility of BAL in patients with idiopathic interstitial pneumonias (IIPs) (group II)

FIBROSING IIPS

Idiopathic pulmonary fibrosis (IPF)

IPF, clinically characterized by progressive scarring in the lungs, is morphologically defined by a UIP pattern, and IPF diagnosis requires the exclusion of other known causes of ILD.

The most common BALF finding in IPF is a variable increase in neutrophils, often accompanied by a minor increase in eosinophils, and occasionally a small increase in lymphocytes not exceeding 30% (12).

However, the role of BAL in the diagnosis of IPF depends on the HRCT pattern (25). If a patient presents with UIP pattern on HRCT, accompanied by a clinical presentation compatible with IPF, BAL is not mandatory according to the recently updated international IPF guideline but can be helpful to exclude other possible ILDs (9).

For example, chronic HP can be indistinguishable from IPF solely based on medical history and radiological findings. Both entities can present with a progressive fibrosing disease course, a UIP HRCT pattern, and the inciting antigen and exposure might not be identified in up to 60% of patients with HP (10, 115, 116). In these cases, a BALF lymphocytosis above the cut-off value of 30% can be a crucial finding to question the diagnosis of IPF.

Conversely, in patients suspected of IPF and presenting with a probable UIP, indeterminate, or alternative HRCT pattern, performing BAL is recommended according to the current IPF guideline (9). When performed, BAL serves mainly to exclude other diseases, particularly those with a lymphocytic or eosinophilic pattern, in the setting of a non-diagnostic HRCT (117). In a study by Ohshimo et al., BALF lymphocytosis (>30%) was found in 6 out of 74 patients with a clinical and radiological diagnosis of IPF, and the final diagnosis in this subgroup of patients revealing BALF lymphocyte levels of >30% was NSIP in three cases and HP in three cases (118).

Another study investigated the role of BAL in patients with indeterminate HRCT patterns. In this subgroup, the presence of BALF lymphocytosis of ≥20% led to a change of diagnosis in 15% of cases, mostly from IPF to chronic HP (119).

Non-specific interstitial pneumonia (NSIP)

NSIP, occurring either as an idiopathic condition or in combination with other known causes including autoimmune diseases, is characterized by bilateral ground-glass opacity as a main finding of HRCT and was first recognized to be a distinct clinical entity in the ATS/ERS international consensus classification of IIPs published in 2013 (2).

The main value of BALF differential cytology findings in the evaluation of patients with suspected NSIP is the identification or exclusion of a predominantly inflammatory cellular pattern (i.e., BALF lymphocytosis) (120). BALF lymphocytosis is observed in cellular NSIP and in mixed patterns of NSIP-OP (121). Indeed, the absence of BALF lymphocytosis has been associated with a diagnosis of IPF rather than of NSIP (OR, 12.7; p < 0.001) (43).

However, the BALF cellular profile of fibrotic NSIP diverges from that of cellular NSIP and shows a cellularity similar to that of IPF, without significant lymphocytosis. Veeraraghavan et al. observed no differences in the clinical profiles (with regard to gender, age, and smoking status) and BALF cellular patterns between fibrotic NSIP and IPF, with neutrophils 9% in both groups, lymphocytes 5% and 4%, respectively, and eosinophils 7% in both groups. Thus, BALF differential cytology might help to differentiate cellular NSIP from IPF, though in the subgroup of fibrotic NSIP, BALF differential cytology findings seem indistinguishable from IPF (122).

SMOKING-ASSOCIATED IDIOPATHIC INTERSTITIAL PNEUMONIAS (IIPS)

In the latest classification of the major IIPs, the term "smoking-related IIP" has been introduced, including DIP and RB-ILD (2).

Radiologically, the most important differential diagnosis of RB-ILD is acute and chronic non-fibrotic HP, which is characterized by centrilobular nodules, ground-glass attenuation, and small airways disease (but not usually bronchial wall thickening) (123). In this situation, the presence of smoker's macrophages and the absence of lymphocytosis suggests the diagnosis of RB-ILD and nearly excludes HP. Thus, in clinical practice, RB-ILD can be diagnosed on the basis of clinical and HRCT findings, complemented by a typical BAL appearance. In contrast to RB-ILD, the diagnostic value of BAL in DIP is limited. BALF findings in DIP typically show an increased cellularity mainly driven by elevated levels of pigmented alveolar macrophages, and a moderate increase in the percentage of eosinophils and neutrophils, but lymphocyte percentages tend to be low (124). Because HRCT findings are also non-characteristic in DIP, histopathological sampling is required for a confident diagnosis of DIP in most cases (125, 126).

ACUTE AND SUBACUTE IIPS

AIP is a rare and fulminant form of diffuse lung injury, formerly known as Hamman and Rich syndrome. AIP is similar in presentation to the acute respiratory distress syndrome (ARDS) and acute exacerbation (AE) of ILD (AE-ILD) and probably represents a subset of cases of idiopathic ARDS. Neutrophil predominance with occasional evidence of hemorrhage related to DAD are the predominant BALF findings (127, 128). Occasionally hyperplastic pneumocytes can also be observed, as in other forms of DAD.

COP, also idiopathic in nature, is characterized by a subacute clinical onset and patchy consolidation on HRCT. BALF findings typically reveal an increased cellularity with a mixed immune cell pattern with variable increases in lymphocytes, neutrophils, eosinophils, and foamy macrophages. Plasma cells and mast cells might be occasionally increased as well (129, 130). Moreover, the CD4+/CD8+ T lymphocyte ratio might be reduced in the BALF of patients of COP, but this finding is variable (130, 131).

Rare IIPs

LIP belongs to the spectrum of benign pulmonary lymphoproliferative disorders. While idiopathic LIP is rare, secondary LIP frequently associated with CTDs or immunodeficiency is more common. A lymphocytic BALF immune cell pattern is the main finding in LIP and a mean lymphocyte differential cell count of 30% was observed in one study including 15 patients with histologically confirmed LIP (132).

Idiopathic PPFE (IPPFE) is a rare fibrosing lung disease, affecting the visceral pleura and the subpleural parenchyma with an upper lobe predilection, included as a distinct clinicopathologic entity in the latest international multidisciplinary classification of the IIP (2).

BALF findings in IPPFE are not specific. In a retrospective case series of nine patients with histologically confirmed IPPFE associated with a UIP HRCT pattern, the BALF cell differential was not different from IPF patients (133).

The diagnostic utility of BAL in patients with granulomatous ILD (group III)

HYPERSENSITIVITY PNEUMONITIS (HP)

HP is a T cell-mediated immunologic lung disease caused by repeated exposure to environmental antigens in susceptible subjects.

A marked lymphocytosis (often >50%) with moderate neutrophilia, modest eosinophilia, and mast cells is the main BALF finding. Foamy macrophages and occasionally plasma cells may also be present (134). A representative photomicrograph of a BALF specimen obtained from a patient with HP is shown in Figure 6.7. A decrease of the CD4$^+$/CD8$^+$ T lymphocyte ratio has been shown to correlate with a diagnosis of HP and might be helpful in differentiating HP from sarcoidosis, but a high variability limits the diagnostic utility of this test in HP (135). The CD4$^+$/CD8$^+$ T lymphocyte ratio might even be increased, especially in patients with chronic HP (46).

In a meta-analysis investigating the findings of 42 studies, which addressed BALF lymphocyte levels in chronic HP, a pooled mean lymphocyte value of 43% was found. In the subgroup of patients with fibrotic HP, the mean lymphocyte value was similarly increased (44%). The percentages of BALF lymphocytes in all other ILD subtypes were lower compared to HP (10% in IPF, 23% in other IIPs, 23% in CTD-ILDs, and 31% in sarcoidosis). A BALF lymphocyte cut-off value of >20% of levels was associated with a sensitivity of 68% and a specificity of 73% to separate between chronic HP and IPF (136). Thus, the magnitude of BALF lymphocytosis has an additional diagnostic value to separate between chronic HP and other fibrotic ILDs (23). BALF lymphocyte cut-off levels of 20–40% have been associated with the best discriminative potential to separate between chronic HP and IPF, even though the optimal cut-off values that define abnormal increases in BALF lymphocyte counts to accurately distinguish HP from other ILDs remain to be determined (123, 137, 138).

With regard to the current ATS/JRS/ALAT clinical practice guideline for the diagnosis of HP in adults, in the case of an identified inciting antigen exposure and/or positive serum IgG testing plus HRCT findings typical for HP (i.e., ground-glass opacity, mosaic attenuation, plus at least one HRCT abnormality suggestive of small airway disease) accompanied by the presence of BALF lymphocytosis, a high-confidence diagnosis of HP (80–89%) can be established even without

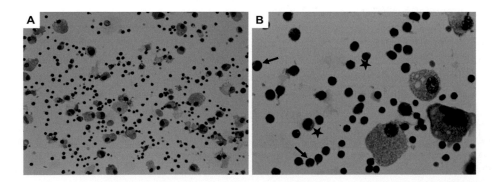

Figure 6.7 (A) A marked lymphocytosis with macrophages characterized by a foamy cytoplasm can be seen in a bronchoalveolar lavage fluid (BALF) sample obtained from a patient with suspected hypersensitivity pneumonitis (May–Grünwald–Giemsa, 200× original magnification). (B) At a higher magnification (600× original magnification), some of the lymphocytes reveal broadened cytoplasm (marked with black arrows) and cleaved nuclei (marked with black stars) as signs of activation.

histopathology sampling, and always after MDD of all findings in the ILD board (123).

According to the CHEST guideline for the diagnosis and evaluation of HP published in 2021, in the same scenario as outlined above – identification of inciting antigen exposure and HRCT findings typical for HP – neither BALF analysis nor histopathology sampling are required to establish a definite HP diagnosis (confidence of ≥90%, also after MDD of the clinical context and HRCT findings). Conversely, in the case of an identified inciting antigen exposure and HRCT findings compatible or indeterminate for HP, the presence of BALF lymphocytosis increases the probability of HP diagnosis from a low-confidence (51–69%) to a high-confidence (70–89%) diagnosis, as compared to the absence of BALF lymphocytosis (138).

SARCOIDOSIS

Sarcoidosis, a multisystem disease of unknown cause characterized by non-caseating granuloma formation mostly affecting the lung, is associated with various clinical phenotypes and heterogenous disease courses.

Although not standardized, the diagnosis of sarcoidosis is based on three major criteria: a compatible clinical presentation, the finding of non-necrotizing granulomatous inflammation in one or more tissue samples, and the exclusion of alternative causes of granulomatous disease. BALF analysis is not required to establish a diagnosis of sarcoidosis, but it can be useful for excluding infections or malignancy or to identify cellular patterns suggestive of eosinophilic lung disease or HP (139).

The most frequent BALF finding in sarcoidosis is a lymphocytosis present in approximately 90% of cases and normal levels of neutrophils and eosinophils, respectively (140). In sarcoidosis, 50–60% of patients reveal an increased CD4$^+$/CD8$^+$ T lymphocyte ratio and a cut-off value of >4 has been shown to be highly specific (specificity ~95%) for a diagnosis of sarcoidosis. However, this ratio can be decreased in up to 15% of patients with sarcoidosis and the CD4$^+$/CD8$^+$ T lymphocyte ratio is not established as a predictor of prognosis or treatment response in sarcoidosis (141).

BERYLLIOSIS

Exposure to beryllium can lead to sensitization (BeS) and CBD. BeS and CBD are the result of a beryllium-specific cell-mediated immune response. A diagnosis of BeS in beryllium-exposed workers undergoing medical surveillance can be based on two abnormal blood beryllium lymphocyte proliferation tests (BeLPTs), one abnormal and one borderline blood BeLPT, or one abnormal BALF BeLPT. Patients with CBD develop a granulomatous inflammation, which is clinically and on imaging similar to sarcoidosis. The main BALF differential cytology finding in CBD is a lymphocytic immune cell pattern as in sarcoidosis. Caution is warranted in smokers and patients with immunosuppression because BALF BeLPTs might reveal false negative results in these patients (142).

The diagnostic utility of BAL in patients with other types of ILD (group IV)

Rare ILD entities are subsumed under this group.

PLCH and LAM are examples of cystic ILDs. When characteristic HRCT findings are accompanied by a typical clinical presentation, a diagnosis of PLCH and LAM can be made without performing BAL or tissue sampling.

In LAM, no specific BALF immune cell patterns have been described, but mild to moderate alveolar hemorrhage might be present (143).

BALF findings in PLCH are often similar to those in smokers and might reveal an increased cellularity with macrophage predominance. A mild or moderate lymphocytosis, slight neutrophilia, or eosinophilia can even be observed, but these findings are inconsistent between studies (65). BALF immune cells demonstrating positivity for CD1a in >5% of cells is a highly specific finding for PLCH; although only ~50% of patients show this elevation of CD1a$^+$ cells (48, 144).

PAP syndrome as well as acute and chronic eosinophilic pneumonia are other rare ILD entities. BALF findings in these diseases are highly characteristic and detailed in the section "Highly specific and pathognomonic BALF findings in ILD" (see also Table 6.3).

THE UTILITY OF PERFORMING BAL IN THE MANAGEMENT OF SELECTED SCENARIOS IN ILD

Acute exacerbation of ILD

AE-ILD, either triggered, e.g., by infection, post-procedural/post-operative, drug toxicity, aspiration, or idiopathic (145), is a frequently fatal complication of IPF and other fibrosing ILDs (146).

As reviewed by Faverio et al., three scenarios should be considered in the management of patients with AE-ILD. First, AE can occur in patients with known chronic ILD. Second, AE can be present in a patient with underlying unknown chronic ILD. Third, AE might be the clinical manifestation of de novo acute ILD or AIP (147).

AE-ILD should be considered as differential diagnosis in the first two scenarios and requires urgent diagnostic management. An international survey including 509 pulmonologists from 66 countries, issuing differences according to the management strategies of AE-IPF, revealed that 5.8% of the responding clinicians always performed BAL, while the majority (70.5%) only performed BAL in case of suspected infection (148).

The role of bronchoscopic assessment of AE-ILD was also elucidated by Arcadu et al. (149). In this retrospective study, 106 consecutive ILD patients who were hospitalized with AE and underwent bronchoscopy were included. Bronchoscopy findings only affected management in 13% of patients and resulted in a change of treatment in less than 5% of patients.

It must be noted that in this study bronchoscopy was associated with an increased risk of endotracheal intubation after the procedure, and a significant number of patients could not be extubated afterwards. Although another study demonstrated the feasibility and safety of BAL aided by non-invasive ventilation for differentiating or confirming triggered AE of ILD (150), these results emphasize the need for a careful risk–benefit analysis before performing BAL in patients with AE-ILD based on an individual case-by-case decision.

Based on the results of two Japanese retrospective cohort studies investigating BALF differential cell count findings in patients with AE-ILD, a lymphocytic, a neutrophilic, and a mixed lymphocytic/neutrophilic cellular pattern was identified.

In the study performed by Takei et al., 37 patients with AE-ILD who underwent BAL were dichotomized into subjects with low lymphocyte levels and high BALF lymphocyte levels based on a lymphocyte cut-off value of 15%. There were no differences with regard to the distribution of HRCT patterns (UIP vs non-UIP HRCT pattern) between both lymphocyte groups (24 subjects had a high BALF lymphocyte count and 13 subjects had a low BALF lymphocyte count), and also BALF neutrophil levels were not associated with a particular HRCT pattern. A lymphocyte differential count >15% in BALF was associated with favorable outcomes (151).

In the study performed by Kono et al., BALF differential cytology findings of 71 patients diagnosed with AE-ILD were correlated with radiographic and clinical findings. BALF neutrophil counts were significantly increased in subjects with an underlying UIP HRCT pattern, and there was a significant negative correlation between BALF neutrophil cell counts and the PaO_2/FiO_2 ratio independent of the underlying HRCT pattern. In 14 patients who underwent BAL in both the stable and AE phases, the percentage of neutrophils in BALF was significantly higher in the AE phase than in the stable phase. BALF lymphocyte and a neutrophil count of $\geq$25% and <20%, respectively, predicted favorable survival after AE (152).

AE has been studied most intensively in IPF. Similar to IPF, HP can also present with a progressive fibrosing disease course and a UIP HRCT pattern, and certain molecular risk factors have been described for both, IPF and chronic HP (e.g., the MUC5B promotor polymorphism and shorter telomere lengths have been associated with the development and risk of progression in both, IPF and chronic HP) (153, 154).

Kang et al. investigated the incidence rate and risk factors of AE and their effect on the survival of 101 patients with histologically confirmed fibrotic HP. During a median follow-up period of 30 months, 33 of the patients developed rapid respiratory deterioration, of which 18 patients fulfilled the criteria of AE, based on the definition criteria previously used in IPF (155). BALF lymphocytosis of >20% was observed in 42% of the included patients. No significant differences regarding BALF total cell counts, BALF neutrophils, and BALF lymphocyte levels were observed between the patient groups (patients with no rapid deterioration (n = 68) vs patients with AE (n = 18) vs patients with other causes of rapid deterioration (n = 15)). BALF differential findings were neither identified as a predictor for the development of AE, nor as a risk factor for all-cause mortality, when included in a multivariable logistic regression model (156).

Miyazaki et al. investigated 100 consecutive patients with chronic HP, of whom 14 patients developed AE, whereas 86 patients remained stable. The mean BALF lymphocyte count at the time of HP diagnosis was lower in the group of patients who developed AE compared to those with a stable disease course. Conversely, the number of neutrophils at the time of HP diagnosis was greater in patients who developed AE than in the group of patients with a stable disease course. The authors concluded that low total lung capacity (TLC) and diffusing capacity of the lung for carbon monoxide (DLco), low BALF lymphocyte levels, and a UIP-like pattern in histology at the time of diagnosis may be the risk factors for AE in patients with chronic HP (157).

Other potentially life-threatening complications in the first two scenarios include purulent infections of the lower respiratory tract, drug reactions, and hemorrhage (see also Table 6.1 and Table 6.3).

If hemorrhage is suspected, serial BAL can be performed to distinguish between blood that originates from an airway lesion potentially associated with active bleeding or being the result of DAH (158). An increase in blood on serial BAL is suggestive of DAH syndrome, which can even be occult.

The third scenario refers mainly to patients with AIP, COP, AEP, and drug-induced ILD. BALF differential cytology findings can be of help to exclude some of these disorders or to narrow the differential diagnosis, as shown in Table 6.1 and Table 6.3.

The role of BAL in patients with progressive pulmonary fibrosis

Although stabilization or improvement of ILD under treatment is possible, 18–32% of cases of fibrotic ILD reveal a progressive phenotype (PF-ILD), despite the current best treatment (159). The term progressive pulmonary fibrosis (PPF) is defined as the presence of at least two of three criteria (worsening symptoms, lung function decline, and radiological progression) occurring within the past year and no alternative explanation in a patient with an ILD other than IPF (9).

Importantly, the term PPF reflects a common disease phenotype of different ILDs and should not be regarded as a distinct ILD entity. BALF cellular analysis is neither an established diagnostic tool in the clinical routine to predict the development of a progressive fibrosing ILD phenotype nor to forecast the risk of disease progression in an individual patient with PPF (160). However, performing BAL in PPF might still be useful to determine the extent of inflammation, e.g., in the case of fibrosing HP (136).

The role of BAL in monitoring disease activity, guiding therapy, and providing prognostic information in patients with ILD

The clinical utility of BALF analyses to assess disease activity, to provide prognostic information, or to guide treatment decisions in ILD was addressed in several research studies.

One potential bias that might affect any of these studies is that for example, UIP and NSIP may coexist in the same patient. In this situation, prognosis was shown to be mainly driven by the pattern associated with the worst outcome (161). If BALF was taken from a lung segment predominantly affected by NSIP, BALF differential cell count might reveal a lymphocytic immune cell pattern. However, prognosis in this case would be largely determined by the UIP pattern, which is typically associated with IPF and a neutrophilic BALF immune cell pattern.

Independent from the underlying histological subtype, BALF lymphocytosis has been associated with a better response to anti-inflammatory therapy and has been correlated with improved outcomes in patients with chronic fibrosing IIPs (43).

As shown by Yamagata et al., BALF lymphocyte differential cell count of >15% has been shown to be a predictive biomarker for identifying patients with fibrotic ILDs who are likely to benefit from anti-inflammatory drugs (92).

In another study, a low BALF lymphocytosis, as defined as the presence of a BALF lymphocyte differential cell count ≤20%, and the presence of honeycombing were predictors of a poor outcome and the absence of corticosteroid (CS) treatment effect in fibrotic HP (93).

Further, a couple of studies suggested that BALF neutrophilia might be associated with a poor prognosis in ILDs associated with UIP and NSIP HRCT or histopathological patterns. BALF neutrophilia for instance was shown to be a predictor of early mortality in IPF and the presence of BALF lymphocytosis correlated with a better prognosis in IPF (162).

Data on the prognostic value of BALF differential cytology findings in AE-ILD are likewise limited.

BALF lymphocytosis predicted a favorable survival in AE-ILD. Moreover, corticosteroids and other immunosuppressants were more effective in patients with AE-ILD when BALF lymphocytosis was present, even though cut-off values for the definition of BALF lymphocytosis varied between studies. In contrast, a BALF neutrophilic cell count of ≥21% cell pattern in AE-ILD was associated with poorer outcomes and CS treatment failure in AE-ILD (151, 152).

In a retrospective analysis investigating 50 patients receiving invasive mechanical ventilation for ARDS with no common risk factors based on the Berlin definition of ARDS (163), increased BALF lymphocyte levels and DAH were associated with an improved intensive care unit (ICU) survival. Of these 50 patients, 18 were diagnosed with CVD, 13 with drug-induced ARDS, 7 had underlying malignancy, and no cause of ARDS could be identified in 12 patients. In the group of survivors (n = 17), the mean BALF lymphocyte count was 66% (inter quartile range (IQR): 11–87) compared to a mean BALF lymphocyte count of 12% (IQR: 5–36) in the group of non-survivors.

Importantly, the ICU mortality did not differ significantly according to the four etiological subgroups (164).

CONCLUSION

BAL is principally indicated in all patients with suspected ILD or unclear pulmonary opacities on chest imaging.

BAL, usually performed during flexible bronchoscopy under conscious sedation, is a safe procedure and can also be performed in critically ill patients requiring non-invasive or invasive ventilatory support.

BALF differential cytology findings can be categorized into different immune cell patterns and the identification or exclusion of each of these patterns is associated with an increased likelihood of certain ILD subtypes. However, these immune cell patterns are not specific but can be of help to narrow the differential diagnosis. For example, BALF lymphocyte levels, though the proposed thresholds varied across studies, can be helpful to distinguish between IPF and chronic fibrotic HP, which can both present with similar HRCT patterns and a progressive fibrosing disease course.

BALF findings can be highly specific, particularly in alveolar-filling processes. The absence of characteristic BALF findings can also be of value to exclude infections, DAH syndrome, or eosinophilic lung diseases.

BALF tests beyond Wright–Giemsa or MGG staining for differential cell cytology include lymphocyte subset analyses either performed by flow cytometry or immunocytochemistry, PAS staining, or ORO staining in the case of suspected PAP syndrome or aspiration, respectively. Hemosiderin staining is indicated in suspected DAH syndrome and the presence of ≥20% hemosiderin-laden macrophages is highly specific for this condition.

It has not been established whether BALF findings are clinically beneficial for assessing disease activity, for providing prognostic information, or for guiding therapy in ILD.

In the future, BALF lymphocyte subset analysis via flow cytometry and/or multiplex immunoassays for cytokine secretion profiling, BALF proteomics, and the identification of ILD endotypes by using next-generation-sequencing based transcriptomic analysis might expand the application spectrum of BALF analysis in ILD to pave the way for a personalized management and targeted therapies for ILD patients.

REFERENCES

1. Agusti C, American Thoracic Society/ European Respiratory Society International multidisciplinary consensus classification of the idiopathic interstitial pneumonias (vol 165, pg 277, 2002). *Am J Resp Crit Care* 2002;166(3):426.

2. Travis WD, Costabel U, Hansell DM, King TE, Jr., Lynch DA, Nicholson AG, et al. An official American Thoracic Society/ European Respiratory Society statement: Update of the international multidisciplinary classification of the idiopathic interstitial pneumonias. *Am J Respir Crit Care Med* 2013;188(6):733–48.

3. Skolnik K, Ryerson CJ. Unclassifiable interstitial lung disease: A review. *Respirology* 2016;21(1):51–6.

4. Maher TM, Bendstrup E, Dron L, Langley J, Smith G, Khalid JM, et al. Global incidence and prevalence of idiopathic pulmonary fibrosis. *Respir Res* 2021;22(1):197.

5. Hutchinson J, Fogarty A, Hubbard R, McKeever T. Global incidence and mortality of idiopathic pulmonary fibrosis: A systematic review. *Eur Respir J* 2015;46(3):795–806.

6. Hilberg O, Hoffmann-Vold AM, Smith V, Bouros D, Kilpelainen M, Guiot J, et al. Epidemiology of interstitial lung diseases and their progressive-fibrosing behaviour in six European countries. *ERJ Open Research* 2022;8(1):00597–2021.

7. Singh S, Collins BF, Sharma BB, Joshi JM, Talwar D, Katiyar S, et al. Interstitial lung disease in India: Results of a prospective registry. *Am J Respir Crit Care Med* 2017;195(6):801–13.

8. Mapel DW, Coultas DB. The environmental epidemiology of idiopathic interstitial lung disease including sarcoidosis. *Semin Resp Crit Care* 1999;20(6):521–9.

9. Raghu G, Remy-Jardin M, Richeldi L, Thomson CC, Inoue Y, Johkoh T, et al. Idiopathic pulmonary fibrosis (an update) and progressive pulmonary fibrosis in adults: An official ATS/ERS/JRS/ALAT clinical practice guideline. *Am J Respir Crit Care Med* 2022;205(9):e18–e47.

10. Fernandez Perez ER, Swigris JJ, Forssen AV, Tourin O, Solomon JJ, Huie TJ, et al. Identifying an inciting antigen is associated with improved survival in patients with chronic hypersensitivity pneumonitis. *Chest* 2013;144(5):1644–51.

11. Drent M, Crouser ED, Grunewald J. Challenges of sarcoidosis and its management. *N Engl J Med* 2021;385(11):1018–32.

12. Meyer KC, Raghu G, Baughman RP, Brown KK, Costabel U, du Bois RM, et al. An official American Thoracic Society clinical practice guideline: The clinical utility of bronchoalveolar lavage cellular analysis in interstitial lung disease. *Am J Resp Crit Care* 2012;185(9):1004–14.

13. Hiwatari N, Shimura S, Takishima T, Shirato K. Bronchoalveolar lavage as a possible cause of acute exacerbation in idiopathic pulmonary fibrosis patients. *Tohoku J Exp Med* 1994;174(4):379–86.

14. Kim DS, Park JH, Park BK, Lee JS, Nicholson AG, Colby I. Acute exacerbation of idiopathic pulmonary fibrosis: Frequency and clinical features. *Eur Respir J* 2006;27(1):143–50.

15. Sakamoto K, Taniguchi H, Kondoh Y, Wakai K, Kimura T, Kataoka K, et al. Acute exacerbation of IPF following diagnostic bronchoalveolar lavage procedures. *Respir Med* 2012;106(3):436–42.

16. Maher TM, Oballa E, Simpson JK, Porte J, Habgood A, Fahy WA, et al. An epithelial biomarker signature for idiopathic pulmonary fibrosis: An analysis from the multicentre PROFILE cohort study. *Lancet Respir Med* 2017;5(12):946–55.

17. Molyneaux PL, Smith JJ, Saunders P, Chua F, Wells AU, Renzoni EA, et al. BAL is safe and well tolerated in individuals with idiopathic pulmonary fibrosis: An analysis of the PROFILE study. *Am J Resp Crit Care* 2021;203(1):136–9.

18. Kondoh Y, Taniguchi H, Kitaichi M, Yokoi T, Johkoh T, Oishi T, et al. Acute exacerbation of interstitial pneumonia following surgical lung biopsy. *Respir Med* 2006;100(10):1753–9.

19. Ravaglia C, Bonifazi M, Wells AU, Tomassetti S, Gurioli C, Piciucchi S, et al. Safety and diagnostic yield of transbronchial lung cryobiopsy in diffuse parenchymal lung diseases: A comparative study versus video-assisted thoracoscopic lung biopsy and a systematic review of the literature. *Respiration* 2016;91(3):215–27.

20. Baughman RP. Technical aspects of bronchoalveolar lavage: Recommendations for a standard procedure. *Semin Resp Crit Care* 2007;28(5):475–85.

21. Mohan A, Madan K, Hadda V, Tiwari P, Mittal S, Guleria R, et al. Guidelines for diagnostic flexible bronchoscopy in adults: Joint Indian chest society/national college of chest physicians (I)/Indian association for bronchology recommendations. *Lung India*. 2019;36:S37–S89.

22. Flaherty KR, King TE, Raghu G, Lynch JP, Colby TV, Travis WD, et al. Idiopathic interstitial pneumonia - What is the effect of a multidisciplinary approach to diagnosis? *Am J Resp Crit Care* 2004;170(8):904–10.

23. Bonella F, Costabel U. The perpetual enigma of bronchoalveolar lavage fluid lymphocytosis in chronic hypersensitivity pneumonitis: Is it of diagnostic value? *Eur Respir J* 2020;56(2).

24. Costabel U, Guzman J, Bonella F, Oshimo S. Bronchoalveolar lavage in other interstitial lung diseases. *Semin Respir Crit Care Med* 2007;28(5):514–24.

25. Raghu G, Remy-Jardin M, Myers JL, Richeldi L, Ryerson CJ, Lederer DJ, et al. Diagnosis of idiopathic pulmonary fibrosis. An official ATS/ERS/JRS/ALAT clinical practice guideline. *Am J Respir Crit Care Med* 2018;198(5):e44–e68.

26. Kebbe J, Abdo T. Interstitial lung disease: The diagnostic role of bronchoscopy. *J Thorac Dis* 2017;9:S996–S1010.

27. Hetzel J, Kreuter M, Kahler CM, Kabitz HJ, Gschwendtner A, Eberhardt R, et al. Bronchoscopic performance of bronchoalveolar lavage in Germany - A call for standardization. *Sarcoidosis Vasc Diffuse Lung Dis* 2021;38(1):e2021003.

28. Haslam PL, Baughman RP. Report of ERS task force: Guidelines for measurement of acellular components and standardization of BAL. *Eur Respir J* 1999;14(2):245–8.

29. Klech H, Pohl W. Technical recommendations and guidelines for bronchoalveolar lavage (BAL). *Eur Respir J* 1989;2(6):561–85.

30. Klech H. Clinical guidelines and indications for bronchoalveolar lavage (BAL) - Report of the European Society of Pneumology task group on BAL - Introduction. *Eur Respir J* 1990;3(8):939.

31. Costabel U. [Recommendations for diagnostic bronchoalveolar lavage. German society of pneumology]. *Pneumologie* 1993;47(11):607–19.

32. Allen JN, Davis WB, Pacht ER. Diagnostic-significance of increased bronchoalveolar lavage fluid eosinophils. *Am Rev Respir Dis* 1990;142(3):642–7.

33. Pope-Harman AL, Davis WB, Allen ED, Christoforidis AJ, Allen JN. Acute eosinophilic pneumonia - A summary of 15 cases and review of the literature. *Medicine* 1996;75(6):334–42.

34. Sitbon O, Bidel N, Dussopt C, Azarian R, Braud ML, Lebargy F, et al. Minocycline pneumonitis and eosinophilia - A report on 8 patients. *Arch Intern Med* 1994;154(14):1633–40.

35. Costabel U, Uzaslan E, Guzman J. Bronchoalveolar lavage in drug-induced lung disease. *Clin Chest Med* 2004;25(1):25–35.

36. Winterbauer RH, Lammert J, Selland M, Wu R, Corley D, Springmeyer SC. Bronchoalveolar lavage cell populations in the diagnosis of sarcoidosis. *Chest* 1993;104(2):352–61.

37. Keogh BA, Hunninghake GW, Line BR, Crystal RG. The alveolitis of pulmonary sarcoidosis - Evaluation of natural-history and alveolitis-dependent changes in lung-function. *Am Rev Respir Dis* 1983;128(2):256–65.

38. Ratjen F, Costabel U, Griese M, Paul K. Bronchoalveolar lavage fluid findings in children with hypersensitivity pneumonitis. *Eur Respir J* 2003;21(1):144–8.

39. Yoshizawa Y, Ohtani Y, Hayakawa H, Sato A, Suga M, Ando M. Chronic hypersensitivity pneumonitis in Japan: A nationwide epidemiologic survey. *J Allergy Clin Immunol* 1999;103(2 Pt 1):315–20.

40. Schnabel A, Richter C, Bauerfeind S, Gross WL. Bronchoalveolar lavage cell profile in methotrexate induced pneumonitis. *Thorax* 1997;52(4):377–9.

41. Akoun GM, Cadranel JL, Milleron BJ, D'Ortho MP, Mayaud CM. Bronchoalveolar lavage cell data in 19 patients with drug-associated pneumonitis (except amiodarone). *Chest* 1991;99(1):98–104.

42. Shimizu S, Yoshinouchi T, Ohtsuki Y, Fujita J, Sugiura Y, Banno S, et al. The appearance of S-100 protein-positive dendritic cells and the distribution of lymphocyte subsets in idiopathic nonspecific interstitial pneumonia. *Respir Med* 2002;96(10):770–6.

43. Ryu YJ, Chung MP, Han J, Kim TS, Lee KS, Chun EM, et al. Bronchoalveolar lavage in fibrotic idiopathic interstitial pneumonias. *Respir Med* 2007;101(3):655–60.

44. Bonella F, Ohshimo S, Bauer P, Guzman J, Costabel U. Bronchoalveolar lavage. In: Strausz J, Bolliger CT, editors. *Interventional Pneumology. European Respiratory Society Monograph. 48.* European Respiratory Society; 2010, pp. 59–72.

45. Costabel U, Bross KJ, Ruhle KH, Lohr GW, Matthys H. Ia-like antigens on T-cells and their subpopulations in pulmonary sarcoidosis and in hypersensitivity pneumonitis - Analysis of bronchoalveolar and blood-lymphocytes. *Am Rev Respir Dis* 1985;131(3):337–42.

46. Barrera L, Mendoza F, Zuniga J, Estrada A, Zamora AC, Melendro EI, et al. Functional diversity of T-cell subpopulations in subacute and chronic hypersensitivity pneumonitis. *Am J Respir Crit Care Med* 2008;177(1):44–55.

47. Meyer KC, Soergel P. Variation of bronchoalveolar lymphocyte phenotypes with age in the physiologically normal human lung. *Thorax* 1999;54(8):697–700.

48. Auerswald U, Barth J, Magnussen H. Value of Cd-1-Positive cells in bronchoalveolar lavage fluid for the diagnosis of pulmonary histiocytosis-X. *Lung* 1991;169(6):305–9.

49. Trapnell BC, Nakata K, Bonella F, Campo I, Griese M, Hamilton J, et al. Pulmonary alveolar proteinosis. *Nat Rev Dis Primers* 2019;5(1):16.

50. Knauer-Fischer S, Ratjen F. Lipid-laden macrophages in bronchoalveolar lavage fluid as a marker for pulmonary aspiration. *Pediatr Pulmonol* 1999;27(6):419–22.

51. Lee AS, Lee JS, He Z, Ryu JH. Reflux-aspiration in chronic lung disease. *Ann Am Thorac Soc* 2020;17(2):155–64.

52. Torous VF, Brackett D, Brown P, Edwin N, Heidarian A, Lobuono C, et al. Oil Red O staining for lipid-laden macrophage index of bronchoalveolar lavage: Interobserver agreement and challenges to interpretation. *J Am Soc Cytopathol* 2020;9(6):563–9.

53. Basset-Leobon C, Lacoste-Collin L, Aziza J, Bes JC, Jozan S, Courtade-Saidi M. Cut-off values and significance of Oil Red O-positive cells in bronchoalveolar lavage fluid. *Cytopathology* 2010;21(4):245–50.

54. Green RJ, Ruoss SJ, Kraft SA, Berry GJ, Raffin TA. Pulmonary capillaritis and alveolar hemorrhage - Update on diagnosis and management. *Chest* 1996;110(5):1305–16.

55. De Lassence A, Fleury-Feith J, Escudier E, Beaune J, Bernaudin JF, Cordonnier C. Alveolar hemorrhage. Diagnostic criteria and results in 194 immunocompromised hosts. *Am J Respir Crit Care Med* 1995;151(1):157–63.

56. Philit F, Etienne-Mastroianni B, Parrot A, Guerin C, Robert D, Cordier JF. Idiopathic acute eosinophilic pneumonia - A study of 22 patients. *Am J Resp Crit Care* 2002;166(9):1235–9.

57. Allen J. Acute eosinophilic pneumonia. *Semin Resp Crit Care* 2006;27(2):142–7.

58. De Giacomi F, Vassallo R, Yi ES, Ryu JH. Acute eosinophilic pneumonia. Causes, diagnosis, and management. *Am J Respir Crit Care Med* 2018;197(6):728–36.

59. Marchand E, Cordier JF. Idiopathic chronic eosinophilic pneumonia. *Orphanet J Rare Dis* 2006;1:11.

60. Crowe M, Robinson D, Sagar M, Chen L, Ghamande S. Chronic eosinophilic pneumonia: Clinical perspectives. *Ther Clin Risk Manag* 2019;15:397–403.

61. Rennard SI. Bronchoalveolar lavage in the diagnosis of cancer. *Lung* 1990;168:1035–40.

62. Chou CW, Lin FC, Tung SM, Liou RD, Chang SC. Diagnosis of pulmonary alveolar proteinosis - Usefulness of Papanicolaou-stained smears of bronchoalveolar lavage fluid. *Arch Intern Med* 2001;161(4):562–6.

63. Lauque D, Dongay G, Levade T, Caratero C, Carles P. Bronchoalveolar lavage in liquid paraffin pneumonitis. *Chest* 1990;98(5):1149–55.

64. Corwin RW, Irwin RS. The lipid-laden alveolar macrophage as a marker of aspiration in parenchymal lung-disease. *Am Rev Respir Dis* 1985;132(3):576–81.

65. Baqir M, Vassallo R, Maldonado F, Yi ES, Ryu JH. Utility of bronchoscopy in pulmonary Langerhans cell histiocytosis. *J Bronchol Interv Pulmonol* 2013;20(4):309–12.

66. Takizawa Y, Taniuchi N, Ghazizadeh M, Enomoto T, Sato M, Jin E, et al. Bronchoalveolar lavage fluid analysis provides diagnostic information on pulmonary Langerhans cell histiocytosis. *J Nippon Med Sch* 2009;76(2):84–92.

67. Grebski E, Hess T, Hold G, Speich R, Russi E. Diagnostic value of hemosiderin-containing macrophages in bronchoalveolar lavage. *Chest* 1992;102(6):1794–9.

68. Ioachimescu OC, Stoller JK. Diffuse alveolar hemorrhage: Diagnosing it and finding the cause. *Cleve Clin J Med* 2008;75(4):258, 60, 64–5 passim.

69. Israel-Biet D, Venet A, Caubarrere I, Bonan G, Danel C, Chretien J, et al. Bronchoalveolar lavage in amiodarone pneumonitis. Cellular abnormalities and their relevance to pathogenesis. *Chest* 1987;91(2):214–21.

70. Coudert B, Bailly F, Lombard JN, Andre F, Camus P. Amiodarone pneumonitis. Bronchoalveolar lavage findings in 15 patients and review of the literature. *Chest* 1992;102(4):1005–12.

71. Ohar JA, Jackson F, Dettenmeier PA, Bedrossian CW, Tricomi SM, Evans RG. Bronchoalveolar lavage cell count and differential are not reliable indicators of amiodarone-induced pneumonitis. *Chest* 1992;102(4):999–1004.

72. Akoun GM, Cadranel JL, Blanchette G, Milleron BJ, Mayaud CM. Bronchoalveolar lavage cell data in amiodarone-associated pneumonitis. Evaluation in 22 patients. *Chest* 1991;99(5):1177–82.

73. Bonella F, Uzaslan E, Guzman J, Costabel C. Bronchoalveolar lavage in drug-induced lung disease. In: *Drug-Induced and Iatrogenic Respiratory Disease*. CRC Press; 2010,pp. 32–42.

74. Hanania AN, Mainwaring W, Ghebre YT, Hanania NA, Ludwig M. Radiation-induced lung injury: Assessment and management. *Chest* 2019;156(1):150–62.

75. Morgan GW, Breit SN. Radiation and the lung: A reevaluation of the mechanisms mediating pulmonary injury. *Int J Radiat Oncol Biol Phys* 1995;31(2):361–9.

76. Nakayama Y, Makino S, Fukuda Y, Min KY, Shimizu A, Ohsawa N. Activation of lavage lymphocytes in lung injuries caused by radiotherapy for lung cancer. *Int J Radiat Oncol Biol Phys* 1996;34(2):459–67.

77. Hoy RF, Chambers DC. Silica-related diseases in the modern world. *Allergy* 2020;75(11):2805–17.

78. DeLight N, Sachs H. *Pneumoconiosis*. Treasure Island (FL): StatPearls; 2022.

79. Vathesatogkit P, Harkin TJ, Addrizzo-Harris DJ, Bodkin M, Crane M, Rom WN. Clinical correlation of asbestos bodies in BAL fluid. *Chest* 2004;126(3):966–71.

80. Wallace JM, Oishi JS, Barbers RG, Batra P, Aberle DR. Bronchoalveolar lavage cell and lymphocyte phenotype profiles in healthy asbestos-exposed shipyard workers. *Am Rev Respir Dis* 1989;139(1):33–8.

81. Karjalainen A, Anttila S, Mantyla T, Taskinen E, Kyyronen P, Tukiainen P. Asbestos bodies in bronchoalveolar lavage fluid in relation to occupational history. *Am J Ind Med* 1994;26(5):645–54.

82. Corhay JL, Delavignette JP, Bury T, Saintremy P, Radermecker MF. Occult exposure to asbestos in steel workers revealed by bronchoalveolar lavage. *Arch Environ Health* 1990;45(5):278–82.

83. Nugent KM, Dodson RF, Idell S, Devillier JR. The utility of bronchoalveolar lavage and transbronchial lung biopsy combined with energy-dispersive X-ray analysis in the diagnosis of silicosis. *Am Rev Respir Dis* 1989;140(5):1438–41.

84. Christman JW, Emerson RJ, Graham WG, Davis GS. Mineral dust and cell recovery from the bronchoalveolar lavage of healthy Vermont granite workers. *Am Rev Respir Dis* 1985;132(2):393–9.

85. Khan SNS, Stirling RG, McLean CA, Russell PA, Hoy RF. GM-CSF antibodies in artificial stone associated silicoproteinosis: A case report and literature review. *Respirol Case Rep* 2022;10(9):e01021.

86. Kayacan O, Beder S, Karnak D. Cellular profile of bronchoalveolar lavage fluid in Turkish miners. *Postgrad Med J* 2003;79(935):527–30.

87. Vallyathan V, Goins M, Lapp LN, Pack D, Leonard S, Shi XL, et al. Changes in bronchoalveolar lavage indices associated with radiographic classification in coal miners. *Am J Resp Crit Care* 2000;162(3):958–65.

88. Antoniou KM, Margaritopoulos G, Economidou F, Siafakas NM. Pivotal clinical dilemmas in collagen vascular diseases associated with interstitial lung involvement. *Eur Respir J* 2009;33(4):882–96.

89. Ng KH, Chen DY, Lin CH, Chao WC, Chen YM, Chen YH, et al. Risk of interstitial lung disease in patients with newly diagnosed systemic autoimmune rheumatic disease: A nationwide, population-based cohort study. *Semin Arthritis Rheum* 2020;50(5):840–5.

90. Tomassetti S, Colby TV, Wells AU, Poletti V, Costabel U, Matucci-Cerinic M. Bronchoalveolar lavage and lung biopsy in connective tissue diseases, to do or not to do? *Ther Adv Musculoskelet Dis* 2021;13:1759720X211059605.

91. Garcia JG, Parhami N, Killam D, Garcia PL, Keogh BA. Bronchoalveolar lavage fluid evaluation in rheumatoid arthritis. *Am Rev Respir Dis* 1986;133(3):450–4.

92. Yamagata A, Arita M, Tachibana H, Tokioka F, Sugimoto C, Sumikawa H, et al. Impact of bronchoalveolar lavage lymphocytosis on the effects of anti-inflammatory therapy in idiopathic non-specific interstitial pneumonia, idiopathic pleuroparenchymal fibroelastosis, and unclassifiable idiopathic interstitial pneumonia. *Respir Res* 2021;22(1):115.

93. De Sadeleer LJ, Hermans F, De Dycker E, Yserbyt J, Verschakelen JA, Verbeken EK, et al. Impact of BAL lymphocytosis and presence of honeycombing on corticosteroid treatment effect in fibrotic hypersensitivity pneumonitis: A retrospective cohort study. *Eur Respir J* 2020;55(4):1901983.

94. Steen VD, Medsger TA. Changes in causes of death in systemic sclerosis, 1972–2002. *Ann Rheum Dis* 2007;66(7):940–4.

95. Hunzelmann N, Genth E, Krieg T, Lehmacher W, Melchers I, Meurer M, et al. The registry of the German Network for Systemic Scleroderma: Frequency of disease subsets and patterns of organ involvement. *Rheumatology (Oxford)* 2008;47(8):1185–92.

96. Cottin V, Brown KK. Interstitial lung disease associated with systemic sclerosis (SSc-ILD). *Respir Res* 2019;20(1):13.

97. Wells AU, Hansell DM, Rubens MB, Cullinan P, Haslam PL, Black CM, et al. Fibrosing alveolitis in systemic-sclerosis - bronchoalveolar lavage findings in relation to computed tomographic appearance. *Am J Resp Crit Care* 1994;150(2):462–8.

98. Goh NS, Veeraraghavan S, Desai SR, Cramer D, Hansell DM, Denton CP, et al. Bronchoalveolar lavage cellular profiles in patients with systemic sclerosis-associated interstitial lung disease are not predictive of disease progression. *Arthritis Rheum* 2007;56(6):2005–12.

99. Kowal-Bielecka O, Kowal K, Highland KB, Silver RM. Bronchoalveolar lavage fluid in scleroderma interstitial lung disease: Technical aspects and clinical correlations: Review of the literature. *Semin Arthritis Rheum* 2010;40(1):73–88.

100. Duarte AC, Porter JC, Leandro MJ. The lung in a cohort of rheumatoid arthritis patients-an overview of different types of involvement and treatment. *Rheumatology (Oxford)* 2019;58(11):2031–8.

101. Hyldgaard C, Hilberg O, Pedersen AB, Ulrichsen SP, Lokke A, Bendstrup E, et al. A population-based cohort study of rheumatoid arthritis-associated interstitial lung disease: Comorbidity and mortality. *Ann Rheum Dis* 2017;76(10):1700–6.

102. Bendstrup E, Moller J, Kronborg-White S, Prior TS, Hyldgaard C. Interstitial lung disease in rheumatoid arthritis remains a challenge for clinicians. *J Clin Med* 2019;8(12):2038.

103. Biederer J, Schnabel A, Muhle C, Gross WL, Heller M, Reuter M. Correlation between HRCT findings, pulmonary function tests and bronchoalveolar lavage cytology in interstitial lung disease associated with rheumatoid arthritis. *Eur Radiol* 2004;14(2):272–80.

104. Gabbay E, Tarala R, Will R, Carroll G, Adler B, Cameron D, et al. Interstitial lung disease in recent onset rheumatoid arthritis. *Am J Respir Crit Care Med* 1997;156(2 Pt 1):528–35.

105. Kowal-Bielecka O, Kowal K, Chyczewska E. Utility of bronchoalveolar lavage in evaluation of patients with connective tissue diseases. *Clin Chest Med* 2010;31(3):423–31.

106. Vuillard C, de Chambrun MP, de Prost N, Guerin C, Schmidt M, Dargent A, et al. Clinical features and outcome of patients with acute respiratory failure revealing anti-synthetase or anti-MDA-5 dermato-pulmonary syndrome: A French multi-center retrospective study. *Ann Intensive Care* 2018;8(1):87.

107. Groen H, Aslander M, Bootsma H, van der Mark TW, Kallenberg CG, Postma DS. Bronchoalveolar lavage cell analysis and lung function impairment in patients with systemic lupus erythematosus (SLE). *Clin Exp Immunol* 1993;94(1):127–33.

108. Wallaert B, Prin L, Hatron PY, Ramon P, Tonnel AB, Voisin C. Lymphocyte sub-populations in bronchoalveolar lavage in Sjogren's syndrome. Evidence for an expansion of cytotoxic/suppressor subset in patients with alveolar neutrophilia. *Chest* 1987;92(6):1025–31.

109. Poletti V, Romagna M, Gasponi A, Baruzzi G, Allen KA. Bronchoalveolar lavage in the diagnosis of low-grade, MALT type, B-cell lymphoma in the lung. *Monaldi Arch Chest Dis* 1995;50(3):191–4.

110. Kadura S, Raghu G. Antineutrophil cytoplasmic antibody-associated interstitial lung disease: A review. *Eur Respir Rev* 2021;30(162):210123.

111. Allen JN, Davis WB. Eosinophilic lung diseases. *Am J Respir Crit Care Med* 1994;150(5 Pt 1):1423–38.

112. Hoffman GS, Sechler JM, Gallin JI, Shelhamer JH, Suffredini A, Ognibene FP, et al. Bronchoalveolar lavage analysis in Wegener's granulomatosis. A method to study disease pathogenesis. *Am Rev Respir Dis* 1991;143(2):401–7.

113. Schnabel A, Reuter M, Gloeckner K, Muller-Quernheim J, Gross WL. Bronchoalveolar lavage cell profiles in Wegener's granulomatosis. *Respir Med* 1999;93(7):498–506.

114. Specks U. Diffuse alveolar hemorrhage syndromes. *Curr Opin Rheumatol* 2001;13(1):12–7.

115. Hanak V, Golbin JM, Ryu JH. Causes and presenting features in 85 consecutive patients with hypersensitivity pneumonitis. *Mayo Clin Proc* 2007;82(7):812–6.

116. Inase N, Ohtani Y, Sumi Y, Umino T, Usui Y, Miyake S, et al. A clinical study of

hypersensitivity pneumonitis presumably caused by feather duvets. *Ann Allergy Asthma Immunol* 2006;96(1):98–104.

117. Raghu G, Richeldi L. Current approaches to the management of idiopathic pulmonary fibrosis. *Respir Med* 2017;129:24–30.

118. Ohshimo S, Bonella F, Cui A, Beume M, Kohno N, Guzman J, et al. Significance of bronchoalveolar lavage for the diagnosis of idiopathic pulmonary fibrosis. *Am J Respir Crit Care Med* 2009;179(11):1043–7.

119. Tzilas V, Tzouvelekis A, Bouros E, Karampitsakos T, Ntasiou M, Katsaras M, et al. Diagnostic value of BAL lymphocytosis in patients with indeterminate for usual interstitial pneumonia imaging pattern. *Eur Respir J* 2019;54(5):1901144.

120. Tomassetti S, Ryu JH, Piciucchi S, Chilosi M, Poletti V. Nonspecific interstitial pneumonia: What is the optimal approach to management? *Semin Respir Crit Care Med* 2016;37(3):378–94.

121. Huo Z, Li J, Li S, Zhang H, Jin Z, Pang J, et al. Organizing pneumonia components in non-specific interstitial pneumonia (NSIP): A clinicopathological study of 33 NSIP cases. *Histopathology* 2016;68(3):347–55.

122. Veeraraghavan S, Latsi PI, Wells AU, Pantelidis P, Nicholson AG, Colby TV, et al. BAL findings in idiopathic nonspecific interstitial pneumonia and usual interstitial pneumonia. *Eur Respir J* 2003;22(2):239–44.

123. Raghu G, Remy-Jardin M, Ryerson CJ, Myers JL, Kreuter M, Vasakova M, et al. Diagnosis of hypersensitivity pneumonitis in adults: An official ATS/JRS/ALAT clinical practice guideline. *Am J Resp Crit Care* 2020;202(3):E36–E69.

124. Kawabata Y, Takemura T, Hebisawa A, Sugita Y, Ogura T, Nagai S, et al. Desquamative interstitial pneumonia may progress to lung fibrosis as characterized radiologically. *Respirology* 2012;17(8):1214–21.

125. Margaritopoulos GA, Harari S, Caminati A, Antoniou KM. Smoking-related idiopathic interstitial pneumonia: A review. *Respirology* 2016;21(1):57–64.

126. Flaherty KR, Fell C, Aubry MC, Brown K, Colby T, Costabel U, et al. Smoking-related idiopathic interstitial pneumonia. *Eur Respir J* 2014;44(3):594–602.

127. Bonaccorsi A, Cancellieri A, Chilosi M, Trisolini R, Boaron M, Crimi N, et al. Acute interstitial pneumonia: Report of a series. *Eur Respir J* 2003;21(1):187–91.

128. Maldonado F, Parambil JG, Yi ES, Decker PA, Ryu JH. Haemosiderin-laden macrophages in the bronchoalveolar lavage fluid of patients with diffuse alveolar damage. *Eur Respir J* 2009;33(6):1361–6.

129. Poletti V, Cazzato S, Minucci N, Zompatori M, Burzi M, Schiattone ML. The diagnostic value of bronchoalveolar lavage and transbronchial lung biopsy in cryptogenic organizing pneumonia. *Eur Respir J* 1996;9(12):2513–6.

130. Costabel U, Teschler H, Guzman J. Bronchiolitis obliterans organizing pneumonia (BOOP): The cytological and immunocytological profile of bronchoalveolar lavage. *Eur Respir J* 1992;5(7):791–7.

131. Cazzato S, Zompatori M, Baruzzi G, Schiattone ML, Burzi M, Rossi A, et al. Bronchiolitis obliterans-organizing pneumonia: An Italian experience. *Respir Med* 2000;94(7):702–8.

132. Cha SI, Fessler MB, Cool CD, Schwarz MI, Brown KK. Lymphoid interstitial pneumonia: Clinical features, associations and prognosis. *Eur Respir J* 2006;28(2):364–9.

133. Oda T, Ogura T, Kitamura H, Hagiwara E, Baba T, Enomoto Y, et al. Distinct characteristics of pleuroparenchymal fibroelastosis with usual interstitial pneumonia compared with idiopathic pulmonary fibrosis. *Chest* 2014;146(5):1248–55.

134. Costabel U, Miyazaki Y, Pardo A, Koschel D, Bonella F, Spagnolo P, et al. Hypersensitivity pneumonitis. *Nat Rev Dis Primers* 2020;6(1):65.

135. Trentin L, Migone N, Zambello R, Dicelle PF, Aina F, Feruglio C, et al. Mechanisms accounting for lymphocytic alveolitis in hypersensitivity pneumonitis. *J Immunol* 1990;145(7):2147–54.

136. Adderley N, Humphreys CJ, Barnes H, Ley B, Premji ZA, Johannson KA. Bronchoalveolar lavage fluid lymphocytosis in chronic hypersensitivity pneumonitis: A systematic review and meta-analysis. *Eur Respir J* 2020;56(2):2000206.

137. Morisset J, Johannson KA, Jones KD, Wolters PJ, Collard HR, Walsh SLF, et al. Identification of diagnostic criteria for chronic hypersensitivity pneumonitis: An international modified Delphi survey. *Am J Respir Crit Care Med* 2018;197(8):1036–44.

138. Perez ERF, Travis WD, Lynch DA, Brown KK, Johannson KA, Selman M, et al. Executive summary diagnosis and evaluation of hypersensitivity pneumonitis: CHEST guideline and expert panel report. *Chest* 2021;160(2):595–615.

139. Crouser ED, Maier LA, Wilson KC, Bonham CA, Morgenthau AS, Patterson KC, et al. Diagnosis and detection of sarcoidosis an official American Thoracic Society clinical practice guideline. *Am J Resp Crit Care* 2020;201(8):E26–E51.

140. Drent M, Mansour K, Linssen C. Bronchoalveolar lavage in sarcoidosis. *Semin Respir Crit Care Med* 2007;28(5):486–95.

141. Costabel U, Bross KJ, Ruhle KH, Lohr GW, Matthys H. Ia-like antigens on T-cells and their subpopulations in pulmonary sarcoidosis and in hypersensitivity pneumonitis. Analysis of bronchoalveolar and blood lymphocytes. *Am Rev Respir Dis* 1985;131(3):337–42.

142. Balmes JR, Abraham JL, Dweik RA, Fireman E, Fontenot AP, Maier LA, et al. An official American Thoracic Society statement: Diagnosis and management of beryllium sensitivity and chronic beryllium disease executive summary. *Am J Resp Crit Care* 2014;190(10):1177–85.

143. Bonetti F, Chiodera PL, Pea M, Martignoni G, Bosi F, Zamboni G, et al. Transbronchial biopsy in lymphangiomyomatosis of the lung - Hmb45 for diagnosis. *Am J Surg Pathol* 1993;17(11):1092–102.

144. Lommatzsch M, Bratke K, Stoll P, Mulleneisen N, Prall F, Bier A, et al. Bronchoalveolar lavage for the diagnosis of pulmonary Langerhans cell histiocytosis. *Respir Med* 2016;119:168–74.

145. Raghu G, Collard HR, Egan JJ, Martinez FJ, Behr J, Brown KK, et al. An official ATS/ERS/JRS/ALAT statement: Idiopathic pulmonary fibrosis: Evidence-based guidelines for diagnosis and management. *Am J Respir Crit Care Med* 2011;183(6):788–824.

146. Song JW, Hong SB, Lim CM, Koh Y, Kim DS. Acute exacerbation of idiopathic pulmonary fibrosis: Incidence, risk factors and outcome. *Eur Respir J* 2011;37(2):356–63.

147. Faverio P, De Giacomi F, Sardella L, Fiorentino G, Carone M, Salerno F, et al. Management of acute respiratory failure in interstitial lung diseases: Overview and clinical insights. *BMC Pulm Med* 2018;18(1):70.

148. Kreuter M, Polke M, Walsh SLF, Krisam J, Collard HR, Chaudhuri N, et al. Acute exacerbation of idiopathic pulmonary fibrosis: International survey and call for harmonisation. *Eur Respir J* 2020;55(4):1901760.

149. Arcadu A, Moua T. Bronchoscopy assessment of acute respiratory failure in interstitial lung disease. *Respirology* 2017;22(2):352–9.

150. Teramachi R, Kondoh Y, Kataoka K, Taniguchi H, Matsuda T, Kimura T, et al. Outcomes with newly proposed classification of acute respiratory deterioration in idiopathic pulmonary fibrosis. *Respir Med* 2018;143:147–52.

151. Takei R, Arita M, Kumagai S, Ito Y, Noyama M, Tokioka F, et al. Impact of lymphocyte differential count > 15% in BALF on the mortality of patients with acute exacerbation of chronic fibrosing idiopathic interstitial pneumonia. *BMC Pulm Med* 2017;17(1):67.

152. Kono M, Miyashita K, Hirama R, Oshima Y, Takeda K, Mochizuka Y, et al. Prognostic significance of bronchoalveolar lavage cellular analysis in patients with acute exacerbation of interstitial lung disease. *Respir Med* 2021;186:106534.

153. Morell F, Villar A, Montero MA, Munoz X, Colby TV, Pipvath S, et al. Chronic hypersensitivity pneumonitis in patients diagnosed with idiopathic pulmonary fibrosis: A prospective case-cohort study. *Lancet Respir Med* 2013;1(9):685–94.

154. Ley B, Newton CA, Arnould I, Elicker BM, Henry TS, Vittinghoff E, et al. The MUC5B promoter polymorphism and telomere length in patients with chronic hypersensitivity pneumonitis: An observational cohort-control study. *Lancet Respir Med* 2017;5(8):639–47.

155. Collard HR, Moore BB, Flaherty KR, Brown KK, Kaner RJ, King TE, Jr., et al. Acute exacerbations of idiopathic pulmonary fibrosis. *Am J Respir Crit Care Med* 2007;176(7):636–43.

156. Kang J, Kim YJ, Choe J, Chae EJ, Song JW. Acute exacerbation of fibrotic hypersensitivity pneumonitis: Incidence and outcomes. *Respir Res* 2021;22(1):152.

157. Miyazaki Y, Tateishi T, Akashi T, Ohtani Y, Inase N, Yoshizawa Y. Clinical predictors and histologic appearance of acute exacerbations in chronic hypersensitivity pneumonitis. *Chest* 2008;134(6):1265–70.

158. Kadar A, Shah VS, Mendoza DP, Lai PS, Aghajan Y, Piazza G, et al. Case 39–2021: A 26-year-old woman with respiratory failure and altered mental status. *N Engl J Med* 2021;385(26):2464–74.

159. Wijsenbeek M, Kreuter M, Olson A, Fischer A, Bendstrup E, Wells CD, et al. Progressive fibrosing interstitial lung diseases: Current practice in diagnosis and management. *Curr Med Res Opin* 2019;35(11):2015–24.

160. Selman M, Pardo A. From pulmonary fibrosis to progressive pulmonary fibrosis: A lethal pathobiological jump. *Am J Physiol-Lung C* 2021;321(3):L600–LL7.

161. Watters LC, Schwarz MI, Cherniack RM, Waldron JA, Dunn TL, Stanford RE, et al. Idiopathic pulmonary fibrosis – Pretreatment bronchoalveolar lavage cellular-constituents and their relationships with lung histopathology and clinical-response to therapy. *Am Rev Respir Dis* 1987;135(3):696–704.

162. Kinder BW, Brown KK, Schwarz MI, Ix JH, Kervitsky A, King TE, Jr. Baseline BAL neutrophilia predicts early mortality in idiopathic pulmonary fibrosis. *Chest* 2008;133(1):226–32.

163. Ranieri VM, Rubenfeld GD, Thompson BT, Ferguson ND, Caldwell E, Fan E, et al. Acute respiratory distress syndrome the Berlin definition. *JAMA* 2012;307(23):2526–33.

164. Gibelin A, Parrot A, Maitre B, Brun-Buisson C, Mekontso Dessap A, Fartoukh M, et al. Acute respiratory distress syndrome mimickers lacking common risk factors of the Berlin definition. *Intensive Care Med* 2016;42(2):164–72.

7

BAL and asthma

PAOLO CAMELI, STEFANO CATTELAN AND MARCO GUERRIERI

Bronchoalveolar lavage (BAL) is a diagnostic procedure that provides relatively easy access to the contents of the lower airways. It consists of instillation and subsequent aspiration of 120–150 ml of saline solution that spreads in the alveoli and distal bronchi. The collected sample can be used to perform microbiological, cytological, ultrastructural, and next-generation analysis tests, including multi-omics assessment (genome, transcriptome, proteome, microbiome, etc.).

It's known that BAL composition can give important information and that this procedure nowadays has a central role in the diagnostic pathway and prognostic estimation of several lung pathologies.

The composition of a healthy individual's BAL is usually characterized by a total cellularity of $100–200 \times 10^3$ cells. Most cells are macrophages, that represent 85–90% of total cells. About 10–12% are lymphocytes. Neutrophils are normally less than 3%. The less-represented cells in the BAL of a healthy patient are basophils and eosinophils (both less than 1%). Squamous epithelial and ciliated columnar epithelial cells contribute to less than 5% of total BAL composition (1). Modifications of these percentages may suggest or even be diagnostic for specific diseases (2).

In recent times, the use of BAL has also been extended to the evaluation and study of small airway disease and in particular to asthma. Even if diagnosis of asthma remains substantially based on clinical features and respiratory functional assessment, BAL may be considered a useful tool to help clinicians in the diagnostic pathway of comorbidities that can contribute to a poor clinical control of asthma, and, therefore, help to a more accurate detection and classification of severe asthma.

In this chapter, beyond the most common respiratory infectious diseases (such as community-acquired pneumonia), we describe the disease entities associated with asthma for which BAL may play a significant role to achieve a diagnosis: allergic broncho-pulmonary aspergillosis (ABPA), eosinophilic pneumonia (EP), bronchiectasis, and eosinophilic granulomatosis with polyangiitis (EGPA).

ALLERGIC BRONCHO-PULMONARY ASPERGILLOSIS

Allergic broncho-pulmonary aspergillosis (ABPA) is an immunological pulmonary disorder caused by hypersensitivity to *Aspergillus fumigatus*. The prevalence of ABPA is about 1–2% in patients with asthma and 2–15% in patients with cystic fibrosis (CF) (3, 4).

The allergic reaction to *Aspergillus* antigens causes a local inflammatory reaction

DOI: 10.1201/9781003146834-9

(characterized by infiltrate of eosinophils, abnormal mucus production, and bronchial wall damage) and an accumulation of mucus plugs, containing *Aspergillus* and eosinophils.

Clinical manifestations can include poorly controlled asthma, wheezing, hemoptysis, and productive cough with expectoration of brownish-black mucus plugs. If untreated, this disease can evolve to pulmonary fibrosis.

Radiologically, chest computed tomography (CT) shows central bronchiectasis, usually involving segmental or subsegmental bronchi, with upper lobe predominance; the presence of high attenuation mucus is a pathognomonic finding of ABPA (5).

Diagnosis is based on clinical, radiological, and laboratory criteria such as hypersensitivity to *Aspergillus fumigatus* (skin test positivity or elevated levels of specific immunoglobulin E (IgE) against *Aspergillus fumigatus* and elevated total IgE levels), presence of typical radiological signs, eosinophilia, and presence of *A. fumigatus* in peripheral blood (6).

Regarding BAL, it can help diagnosis by identifying *Aspergillus* through direct examination and culture. Further, as for serum, *Aspergillus* antigens (galactomannan) and *A. fumigatus* DNA (by polymerase chain reaction [PCR] assays) can be detected in BAL (7).

EOSINOPHILIC PNEUMONIA

Eosinophilic pneumonia (EP) is a rare disorder that includes two major types: acute eosinophilic pneumonia (AEP) and chronic eosinophilic pneumonia (CEP). Both are characterized by a marked accumulation of eosinophils in lung tissues and/or BAL fluid (BALF) (6).

AEP is an idiopathic disease and its etiopathogenesis is still unclear. However, several studies suggest a possible association between AEP onset and smoking habits, such as newly starting smoking or alterations in existing smoking habits, or short-term exposure to passive smoking (8–10). Its association with allergic diseases such as bronchial asthma, dermatitis, and rhinitis is uncommon (less than 10% of cases) (6).

Generally, AEP affects males between 20 and 40 years and it is characterized by acute onset of dyspnea with cough and fever, and it can lead also to an expiratory failure. Usually, it's limited to the lung and doesn't involve other organs. CT shows bilateral pulmonary infiltrates, ground glass opacity, septal thickening, and pleural effusion. Also, CEP is an idiopathic pathology that involves the lung. Even if the cause is not understood, it's known that important factors implicated in asthma (IL-4, IL-5, IL-13, and IgE) are significant elements in its pathogenesis. In fact, a close association between CEP and allergic diseases has been reported, and more than half of patients with CEP have an allergic disease, such as bronchial asthma, atopic dermatitis, and allergic rhinitis (11).

The typical age of onset ranges from the fourth to sixth decades, and symptoms consist of acute or sub-acute onset of progressive dyspnea and productive cough for 1–6 months (12).

Radiological findings include bilateral basal consolidations at CT, while nodules, ground glass opacities, and pleural effusion are less common.

There are no guidelines for the diagnosis of AEP and CEP. For both diseases, it's important the exclusions of secondary causes and the presence of clinical, radiological, and laboratory features compatible with these pathologies.

However, the most important characteristic is represented by the presence of alveolar eosinophilia (eosinophils >25%) that is pathognomonic of EP. For this reason, BAL has a pivotal role in establishing a diagnosis.

EOSINOPHILIC GRANULOMATOSIS WITH POLYANGIITIS

Eosinophilic granulomatosis with polyangiitis (EGPA), previously called Churg–Strauss syndrome (CSS), is a disseminated necrotizing vasculitis with extravascular granulomas occurring in patients with asthma and tissue eosinophilia (13).

The estimated incidence is approximately 0.11 to 2.66 new cases per 1 million people per year, with an overall prevalence of 10.7 to 14 per 1 million adults (14).

EGPA can involve various tissues, but the most common sites are the lung, skin, and nervous system. Diagnosis of this pathology is based on clinical symptoms that can be related to EGPA and typical histopathological findings in biopsy. Rarely, the chosen site for the biopsy is the lung.

Lung histological alterations that could be found in EGPA patients are eosinophilic pneumonia, granulomatous inflammation, and vasculitis. These features could not be present at the same time, so the histological alterations have always been related to clinical symptoms for the diagnosis.

Antineutrophil cytoplasmic antibodies (ANCA) have been found in patients with this pathology and EGPA is part of ANCA-associated vasculitis (AAV) together with granulomatosis with polyangiitis (GPA, Wegener granulomatosis) and microscopic polyangiitis (MPA).

Besides this, hypereosinophilia is one of the main characteristics of this pathology. Thus, EGPA is classified as one of the small-vessel vasculitis associated with ANCAs and as one of the hypereosinophilic syndromes (HESs).

In EGPA, blood eosinophil counts do not necessarily reflect the degree of tissue eosinophilia. It was found that eosinophilia in the BALF can persist in patients with EGPA despite treatment with glucocorticoids, while blood eosinophil count is suppressed effectively.

Trying to better understand the pathogenesis, other studies tried to investigate the mechanism of lung disease due to EGPA, searching the inflammatory cells that can be found in the lower respiratory tract and their BALF levels (15).

Eosinophilic cationic protein (ECP, a protein that is a product of the degranulation of eosinophilic cells) serum level can be high in patients with active EGPA. A high level of this protein has also been found in the BALF of EGPA patients and this demonstrated that eosinophils are active not only systemically, but especially in the site of inflammation. Besides this, activated eosinophils also produce other proteins that are responsible for the tissue and endothelial cell damage, such as major basic protein (MBP) and eosinophil derived neurotoxin (EDN). Another protein that has been detected in the BALF of EGPA patients is myeloperoxidase (MPO), a protein that derives from the degranulation of neutrophilic cells. However, a strict correlation between ECP and MPO levels has not been found, which suggests that eosinophil and neutrophil activation vary independently from each other.

Anyway, it's clear that an eosinophilic population is predominant in the BALF of EGPA patients, and that the neutrophilic cells are less represented.

BRONCHIECTASIS

Non-cystic fibrosis (nCF) bronchiectasis is a condition in which bronchi are irreversibly dilatated and this leads to frequent infection of the lower respiratory airways. Patients with nCF bronchiectasis suffer chronic sputum and bacterial colonization.

Exacerbations of nCF bronchiectasis are defined as a worsening of the symptoms, such as increase in cough (and sputum), wheezing, shortness of breath, hemoptysis, and decline in lung function.

The most important pathogenetic mechanism of exacerbation of nCF bronchiectasis is represented by the role of inflammation of the dilated bronchi that facilitates infections that further perpetuates and worsens the flogistic burden.

Recurrent exacerbations can lead to progressive deterioration of lung function.

Bronchiectasis has been observed in many asthma patients (16) and the presence of asthma is associated with an increased risk in bronchiectasis exacerbation in patients with nCF bronchiectasis (17). Another important factor that increases the risk of exacerbation in patients with bronchiectasis is the presence of *Pseudomonas aeruginosa*.

Fiberoptic bronchoscopy use in patients with nCF bronchiectasis is generally limited. In fact, it's usually recommended to collect sputum for cultural exams. Anyway, bronchoscopy and BAL are recommended in patients in which there's a single lobe involved in the bronchiectasic process and in patients who are not able to produce sputum or in which sputum cultural exams result negative.

Despite this, BAL has a central role in patients with nCF bronchiectasis in finding pathogens that are involved in the infection, especially in defining the presence of *Pseudomonas aeruginosa*. Another infection that is common in patients with nCF bronchiectasis, for which bronchoscopy and BAL can play a central diagnostic role and is a non-tuberculous mycobacterial disease (18). Finding the pathogens involved in nCF bronchiectasis has an important prognostic role and may allow an eradication therapy.

SAFETY OF BAL IN ASTHMA PATIENTS

In the last four decades, fiberoptic bronchoscopy with endobronchial biopsy (EBB) or BAL has been performed in asthma primely for differential diagnosis and also for clinical and translational research. This helped to study the role of inflammation in asthma, studying the morphological and activity features of bronchoalveolar cells and the concentration of inflammatory mediators contributing to the pathogenesis (19). However, BAL safety issues in asthmatic subjects are not to be underestimated: bronchoscopy may lead to a remarkable fall in forced expiratory volume in the first second (FEV1) and asthmatics appeared to experience a more pronounced reduction than other patients (20). Moreover, BAL has been reported as one of the endoscopic procedures more at risk of this issue (21, 22). Thus, although asthma is not considered an absolute or relative contraindication for BAL, the optimization of asthma control is recommended and also nebulized bronchodilators may be considered to be used before the procedure (23).

In 2004 the available data from six studies regarding the safety of bronchoscopy procedures in patients with asthma were collected, for a total of 273 bronchoscopies, 228 of these with EBB and BAL and the remaining 45 EBB alone (24). All recruited patients had a clinical history of asthma: the authors observed that bronchoscopy, including BAL and EBB, has an acceptable profile risk in mild and moderate asthma patients and that most adverse events were mild. Two of the 159 patients had pneumonitis after bronchoscopy, that presented with pleuritic chest pain and fever. Similar results have also been obtained in patients with severe asthma (21). Some authors also suggest that children with severe asthma can tolerate bronchoscopy, but the BAL procedure should be avoided in children with tracheobronchomalacia or current asthma symptoms (25).

PRINCIPAL LINES OF RESEARCH OF BAL IN ASTHMA

Asthma is caused by specific and non-specific irritating stimuli which lead to an inappropriate inflammatory response generating bronchoconstriction, airway remodeling, mucus hypersecretion, and airway hyperreactivity (AHR). In the majority of cases, especially in those affected by a severe disease, the pathogenesis of asthma is sustained by type 2 inflammation, characterized by an aberrant activity of type 2 cells, including lymphocytes, innate lymphoid cells (ILC), eosinophils, mast cells, and B cells (26–29).

Knowledge of the pathogenesis of asthma has been significantly improved thanks to numerous studies in which BAL has been implemented. In fact, BAL represents an important tool to investigate cellular pools and mediators of inflammation of the lower respiratory tract of asthmatic patients, leading to a better understanding of pathogenesis and possible therapeutic target of this condition.

First of all, the analysis of total cell number in BAL of allergic and non-allergic asthmatic subjects shows a higher number of cells than healthy individuals with an increase of percentage of eosinophils (approximately at 2–2.5%) (30–32).

Regarding other mediators of inflammation, it's known that the mast cell population can also be found to have increased in BAL of both atopic and non-atopic asthmatic subjects (33).

Several studies, based on allergen stimulation of atopic patients, demonstrated a high BAL fluid concentration of IL-13 and IL-4. Moreover, in these patients, allergen instillation induces production of pro-inflammatory cytokines (IL-6) and immune modulating cytokines (IL-2, IFN-γ, and IL-10) along with an increased number of lymphocytes and suppressor cells (T-regs and MDSC). Besides this, the allergen challenge shows a significant increase in plasmacytoid dendritic cells (pDC), confirming the crucial role of innate immunity in asthma pathology (34, 35).

BAL cellular analysis may also provide interesting pathogenic insights in specific phenotypes of disease, such as occupational asthma: the exposure to toluene 2,4-diisocyanate (TDI) was reported to significantly increase the BAL concentration of eosinophils, ILC2, and CD4+ lymphocytes in a murine model, supporting the hypothesis that inhalation of TDI may trigger a type2-inflammatory pathway, with relevant clinical insights in terms of clinical management and treatment (36).

The BAL cellular distribution is also influenced by the degree of severity of the disease, since severe asthmatic subjects are associated with lower percentages of BAL monocytes/macrophages, counterbalanced by a higher proportion of neutrophils with respect to mild-to-moderate clinical courses.

According to the evolution of the classification of asthma of the last decades, the analysis of BAL cytokine expression has also confirmed the existence of different inflammatory endotypes: as opposed to allergic and/or eosinophilic, BAL from neutrophilic asthmatic patients showed an enhancement of Th17 and Th1 cytokines, such as IL-17, IL-6, IL-12, and TNF-α (38).

Furthermore, the increase of thymic stromal lymphopoietin (TSLP) BAL concentration is associated with a sustained steroid resistance of type 2 ILCs, leading to reduced effectiveness of corticosteroid treatment in clinical terms (39).

The implementation of flow cytometry analyses has further provided new insights in the pathogenesis of asthma and the differentiation of phenoendotypes of disease. As well as in blood, the differential expression of cell subtypes appeared to be linked to specific features of disease: for example, CD45RO+ ILC2 cells are associated with steroid resistance and a more severe asthma (40), while the imbalance of natural killer (NK) cells subtypes was correlated with worse clinical control and lung function, evaluated through FEV1 (41).

Moreover, BAL cell flows cytometric analysis revealed that ILC proliferation, activity, and expression of surface markers may significantly change over time, localization, and stimulation by different molecules (including alarmins, such as TSLP or IL-33) or allergen stimuli, further underlining the biological complexity of asthma (42).

BAL can be used also to detect the activity of matrix metalloproteinase (MMP)-9 and tissue inhibitor of metalloproteinase (TIMP)-1, very important enzymes involved in the metabolism of the ECM and implicated in tissue remodeling (43).

The chronic inflammation typical of this disease causes damage and metaplasia of the respiratory epithelium; stimulated epithelial cells express large quantities of cytokines/chemokines and metalloproteinases that contribute to an important structural transformation, which affect the airways and leads to their significant functional impairment (44).

Several studies demonstrate elevated MMP-9 a TIMP-1 in blood, sputum, and BAL of asthmatic patients, especially in the atopic ones (45–47).

Detection of the activity of this enzyme may also be useful for clinical practice; in fact, seems that the ratio of sputum MMP-9/TIMP-1 has a positive correlation with the forced expiratory volume in one second (FEV1) of asthmatic patients (48).

Moreover, levels of MMP can also be detected to evaluate the effectiveness of biological therapy with omalizumab in atopic asthma and changing in mediators of inflammation in distal airways after the use of this monoclonal antibody. Omalizumab is associated with a decrease in MMPs in BAL (49).

This depletion is associated with lower inflammation with decreased mucus production, decreased collagen, less proliferation of airway epithelium, smooth muscle hypertrophy, and airway spasm. It results in a reduction in the asthma exacerbation rate and with better asthma controls the inflammation was significantly decreased (50).

In recent years, the implementation of -omics sciences for BAL, associated with next-generation sequencing techniques and artificial intelligence (AI)-powered medical technologies for analysis of big data and the following development of machine-learning models, has contributed to improving the comprehension of biomolecular and immunological mechanisms of asthma. A machine-learning approach applied to the study of BAL cytokine pattern from a big cohort of severe asthmatic subjects was found to discriminate four different phenotypes of disease associated with specific clinical or immunological features (eosinophilic or neutrophilic inflammation, bronchial hyperreactivity, and responsiveness to β2-agonists) (51).

Using the same approach, other clinical features (such as steroid resistance) have been related to a higher BAL expression of IL-4+ innate immune cells and IFN-γ+ T cells and a lower percentage of IL-10+ macrophages (52).

Moreover, the severity of asthma and inflammation clusters associated with different phenoendotypes of disease appeared to be strictly related to the gene expression of resident cells in lower airways, that can be sampled through BAL: in particular, besides age, sex, and cell proportions, the severity of disease was found to be associated with c-AMP signaling: interestingly, medications (such as β2-agonists) are reported to modify cell gene expression, even if the clinical consequences are still to be determined (37).

Interestingly, as for ILC surface markers and activity, a divergent gene expression was reported between BAL and bronchial tissue samplings as well; in particular, IL-13 activity was significantly related to IL-5 and IL-4 in bronchial biopsy and BAL, respectively, suggesting different pathological pathways across respiratory compartments (53).

This assumption was also partially confirmed by the analysis of transcriptome, in which gene expression and transcriptional activity of BAL was not concordant to epithelial and sputum (54).

The transcriptional profile in BAL is also significantly influenced by exposure to specific irritants or allergens, that caused a differential transcriptional response (55).

Finally, the proteomic and lipidomic analysis of BAL fluid have also provided interesting new insights into disease pathogenesis and, potentially, new treatment targets. BAL of asthmatic patients showed a significant increase of oxidative stress markers expression (including chitinases and surfactant protein-D) and a relevant imbalance of galectins, whose levels were associated with eosinophils and fibroblasts presence (56, 57).

Asthma was also associated with an increased airway exosome concentration, correlated with other widely recognized severity biomarkers such as blood eosinophilia and serum IgE levels; furthermore, lipidomics analysis of extracellular vesicles showed many significant modifications of many lipid mediators in respect of healthy controls, leading to a relevant imbalance of phosphatidylglycerol, ceramide-phosphates, ceramides, and sphingomyelin 34:1 exosome expression (58).

REFERENCES

1. Meyer, KC et al., *American Journal of Respiratory and Critical Care Medicine* (2013). PMID: 22550210
2. Harbeck RJ, *Clinical and Diagnostic Laboratory Immunology* (1998). PMID: 9605975
3. Agarwal R, *Chest* (2009). PMID: 19265090
4. Chabi ML et al., *Diagnostic and Interventional Imaging* (2015). PMID: 25753544
5. Agarwal R et al., *Clinical and Experimental Allergy* (2013). PMID: 23889240
6. Suzuki Y et al., *Allergology Interventional: Official Journal of the Japanese Society of Allergology* (2019). PMID: 31253537
7. Lestrade APP et al., *Clinical Microbiology and Infection: The Official Publication of the European Society of Clinical Microbiology and Infectious Diseases* (2018). PMID: 30580035
8. Uchiyama H et al., *Chest* (2008). PMID: 18263675
9. Shorr AF et al., *JAMA* (2004). PMID: 15613668
10. Philit F et al., *American Journal of Respiratory and Critical Care Medicine* (2002). PMID: 12403693
11. Marchand E et al., *Medicine (Baltimore)* (1998). PMID: 9772920
12. Alam M et al., *Southern Medical Journal* (2007). PMID: 17269525
13. Katzenstein ALA, *American Journal of Clinical Pathology* (2000). PMID: 11068552

14. Greco A et al., *Autoimmunity Reviews* (2015). PMID: 25500434
15. Schnabel A et al., *Thorax* (1999). PMID: 10456969
16. Crimi C et al., *Respiration* (2020). PMID: 32464625
17. Mao B et al., *The European Respiratory Journal* (2016). PMID: 27076584
18. Mehdi M et al., *International Journal of Infectious Diseases* (2013). PMID: 23683809
19. Barber C et al., *European Respiratory Journal* (2016). DOI: 10.1183/13993003
20. Van Vyve T et al. *The American Review of Respiratory Disease* (1992). PMID: 1626794
21. Moore WC et al., *The Journal of Allergy and Clinical Immunology* (2011). PMID: 21496892
22. Kariyawasam HH et al., *Thorax* (2007). PMID: 17536034
23. Du Rand IA et al. *Thorax* (2013). PMID: 2386034
24. Elston WJ et al., *European Respiratory Journal* (2004). PMID: 15358694
25. Ben Tkhayat R et al., *European Respiratory Journal* (2021). PMID: 34881325
26. Cohn L et al., *Annual Review of Immunology* (2004). PMID: 15032597
27. Umetsu DT et al., *Nature Immunology* (2002). PMID: 12145657
28. Asquith KL et al., *Journal of Immunology* (2008). PMID: 18178860
29. Holgate ST, *Nature Medicine* (2012). PMID: 22561831
30. Smith DL et al., *American Review of Respiratory Disease* (1993). PMID: 8342920
31. Kim CK et al., *The Journal of Allergy and Clinical Immunology* (2003). PMID: 12847481
32. Kim CK et al., *The Journal of Pediatrics* (2000). PMID: 11035831
33. Casale TB et al., *Journal of Clinical Investigation* (1987). PMID: 3549781
34. Batra V et al., *Journal of the British Society for Allergy and Clinical Immunology* (2004). PMID: 15005738
35. Boomer JS et al., *Allergy, Asthma and Clinical Immunology: Official Journal of the Canadian Society of Allergy and Clinical Immunology* (2013). PMID: 24330650
36. Blomme EE et al., *The European Respiratory Journal* (2020). PMID: 32499335
37. Weathington N et al., *American Journal of Respiratory and Critical Care Medicine* (2019). PMID: 31161938
38. Steinke JW et al., *The Journal of Allergy and Clinical Immunology* (2020). PMID: 32526308
39. Liu S et al., *The Journal of Allergy and Clinical Immunology* (2020). PMID: 28433687
40. Van der Ploeg EK et al., *Science Immunology* (2021). PMID: 33514640
41. Duvall MG et al., *Science Immunology* (2017). PMID: 28783702
42. Li BWS et al., *Frontiers in Immunology* (2017). PMID: 29250067
43. Hrabec E et al., *Postepy Biochemii* (2007). PMID: 17718386
44. Sohal SS et al., *Archivium immunologiae et Therapiae Experimentalis* (2016). PMID: 26123447
45. Gagliardo R et al., *Pediatric Allergy and Immunology: Official Publication of the European Society of Pediatric Allergy and Immunology* (2009). PMID: 19788537
46. Erlewyn-Lajeuness M et al., *Pediatric Research* (2008). PMID: 18391843
47. Ko FWS et al., *Chest* (2005). PMID: 15947303
48. Vignola AM et al., *American Journal of Respiratory and Critical Care Medicine* (1998). PMID: 9847290
49. Zastrzeżyńska W et al., *Journal of Asthma* (2021). PMID: 33764254
50. Korzh O et al., *Journal of Allergy and Clinical Immunology* (2007). DOI: 10.1016/j.jaci.2006.11.542
51. Brasier AR et al., *Clinical and Translational Science* (2010). PMID: 20718815
52. Camiolo MJ et al., *Cells Report* (2021). PMID: 33852838

53. Li X et al., *The Journal of Asthma: Official Journal of the Association for the Care of Asthma* (2016). PMID: 27050946

54. Singhania A et al., *American Journal of Respiratory Cell and Molecular Biology* (2018). PMID: 28933920

55. Yang IV et al., *American Journal of Respiratory and Critical Care Medicine* (2012). PMID: 22246175

56. Zhang L et al., *Journal of Proteome Research* (2009). PMID: 19714806

57. Cederfur C et al., *Biochimica et Biophysica Acta* (2012). PMID: 22240167

58. Hough KP et al., *Scientific Reports* (2018). PMID: 29985427

8

BAL in chronic obstructive pulmonary disease

PARMINDER SINGH BHOMRA, DANIELLA SPITTLE, AND
ALICE M TURNER

INTRODUCTION

Chronic obstructive pulmonary disease (COPD) is a respiratory disease commonly caused by smoking. It is characterized by features throughout the respiratory tract, but predominantly in the small and distal airways. Mucous gland hyperplasia, which occurs particularly in the large airways, along with squamous metaplasia and loss of cilial function leads to mucous hypersecretion and lack of expectoration leading to chronic cough. Chronic inflammation and fibrosis of the small airways mediated by the release of pro inflammatory cytokines produces increased airflow resistance, coupled with emphysema, which is the destruction of alveolar walls distal to the terminal bronchiole causing small airway collapse leading to airflow obstruction. This is demonstrated in Figure 8.1.

Typical symptoms of COPD include shortness of breath, chronic cough (which may be productive), and wheezing. A combination of the above three contributes to a reduction of exercise tolerance and quality of life thereafter. Current treatment is guided by a multidisciplinary approach (1). Medically, there is control of airflow obstruction using inhaled bronchodilator therapy, which when accompanied by features of inflammation such as eosinophilia and reversibility/variability can be combined with inhaled corticosteroids. Pulmonary rehabilitation is a commonly recommended therapeutic intervention to increase exercise tolerance in those patients whose Medical Research Council (MRC) dyspnoea score is 2 and above. Smoking cessation has been shown to reduce the smoking-related decline in lung function and should be recommended to every patient with COPD who continues to smoke, at every opportunity. Surgical options for treatment of COPD include lung transplantation in patients who are deemed eligible by local criteria, bullectomy, and lung volume reduction surgery.

DOI: 10.1201/9781003146834-10

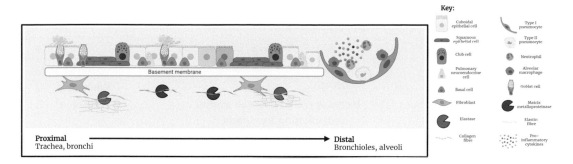

Figure 8.1 Pathophysiology of the large and small airways in COPD. Characteristic changes are present in the epithelial lining throughout the airways of people with COPD. Squamous epithelial cells without cilia populate the proximal COPD airways and mucus-secreting goblet cells are found in higher numbers, compared to those without COPD. Cytokine-secreting innate immune cells (namely, neutrophils and alveolar macrophages) are found in abundance within the distal airways and contribute to local inflammation. Elastase and matrix metalloproteinases contribute to the pathophysiology of COPD by breaking down elastin and collagen within the distal airways, respectively.

CURRENT USE OF BRONCHOSCOPY IN COPD

The role of bronchoscopy in COPD is currently based around excluding alternative diagnoses or investigating recurrent infections in COPD patients who do not produce sputum spontaneously. As an example, if a patient presents with changes of interstitial lung disease (ILD) on a computed tomography (CT) scan, but with features of COPD clinically, BAL can be used for differential cell count in the investigation of ILD. There is currently no role for bronchoscopy in clinical guidelines for the diagnosis of COPD, which is made primarily with clinical features combined with pulmonary function testing and radiology. If there are patients with recurrent infections, or suspicion of an opportunistic infection in someone who is not producing sputum, bronchoscopy for simple bronchial washings can be used as an investigation. The other common situation for bronchoscopy in COPD is in the investigation of lung cancer.

The procedure of BAL specifically is not currently used in clinical practice for COPD and is largely employed for research purposes. As the full pathophysiology of COPD is still not understood, BAL is used frequently in both scientific studies and clinical trials to look at the alveolar environment and the effect of different treatments, given its representation of the distal airways. BAL is often considered a reference standard, particularly in investigations where pharyngeal contamination may perturb findings.

The use of differential cell count, as in the diagnosis of ILD, is still being researched for COPD. However, there seem to be some suggestions of correlation with phenotype. This is addressed later in the chapter.

SAFETY OF BRONCHOSCOPY AND BAL FOR USE IN COPD RESEARCH

The use of bronchoscopy in COPD is considered safe. There are no international guidelines on the use of bronchoscopy specific to COPD. However, the British Thoracic Society (BTS) guidelines for the use of bronchoscopy in COPD recommends the optimization of COPD prior to bronchoscopy and careful use of sedation in COPD patients (2). There have been multiple studies into the safety of BAL in COPD research showing it is safe to use, but the airway characteristics during bronchoscopy, demographic of the patient, and lung function may increase the risk of procedure-related events necessitating intervention, as summarized in Table 8.1 (3–6). Bellinger et al. showed that severe to very severe COPD patients had more

Table 8.1 The table demonstrates how certain clinical, airway and pulmonary function features will increase the risk of bronchoscopy in patients with COPD

COPD feature	Risk with bronchoscopy	Reference
Presence of COPD	Increase in post procedural shortness of breath	Leiten et al. (3) Wells et al. (4)
Increased bronchial secretions	Increase risk of adverse events necessitating treatment*	Wells et al. (4)
Increased airway friability	Increased risk of adverse events necessitating treatment	Wells et al. (4)
Severe to very severe COPD by GOLD classification	Increased risk of respiratory complications**	Bellinger et al. (6)

*Features of COPD and risk with bronchoscopy. Both Leiten et al. and Wells et al. did not include COPD patients with severe disease, such as those with FEV_1 less than 30%, type 2 respiratory failure, or chronic hypoxia. * Adverse events included FEV_1 less than 90% from baseline, failing to meet discharge criteria, chest discomfort, reduced alertness, disorientation, tachycardia, difficulty ambulating, cough/difficulty with sipping water, and admission overnight. ** Respiratory complications included transient desaturation, bronchospasm, epistaxis, transient hypotension, respiratory failure, pneumothorax, and hemoptysis requiring observation.*

complications compared to others (6). As shown in Table 8.1, both Leiten and Wells did not include COPD patients with severe or very severe obstruction, which may suggest that the inclusion of this cohort of patients as seen in Bellinger et al.'s study could show an increase in the risk of respiratory complications/adverse events compared to those without COPD (3, 4). Leiten et al. showed 1.3% of COPD patients had serious complications post research BAL; however, none of these patients developed long-term sequelae (3). They comment on a significant number of patients suffering discomfort post BAL, but these symptoms were tolerable and therefore concluded that BAL is safe to use in COPD research. A combination of the above papers highlights the importance of careful selection of patients in both research and clinical practice for bronchoscopy and BAL in COPD, but ultimately that it appears to be safe.

TECHNICAL DIFFICULTIES OF BAL IN COPD

The use of BAL in COPD varies in research. The amount of fluid infiltrated varies throughout multiple research trials using BAL as an investigative tool. Volumes can be 40–250 ml, with the average being 100–150 ml. We have found variation in the use of the term "bronchoalveolar lavage" in the literature, with some authors labeling 40 ml instillation as a BAL, which may be considered as a simple bronchial wash to others. What is clear, however, is that the percentage yield of bronchoalveolar lavage fluid (BALF) is reduced in patients with COPD (7, 8). In Lofdahl's study looking at BALF recovery in comparison to the degree of emphysema, the median volume of BALF instilled was 245 ml in COPD patients with a 32% median fluid recovery, which was significantly reduced compared to non-smokers where a median of 250 ml fluid was instilled with a 67% recovery (8). Overall, it makes the reliance on BALF difficult as the reduced yield may not be repeatable and therefore not applicable in clinical practice.

A lower recovery of BALF suggests a loss of large amounts of instilled fluid down the small airways. Hence, the majority of fluid recovered and analyzed is likely to be large airway sampling, rather than the alveolar environment. As described in the introduction, the larger airways are not considered to play a primary role in the pathophysiology of COPD and sampling of the large airways is not indicative of the alveolar environment, therefore it may not be an indication for the use of BAL going forward. Lofdahl et al. showed that increasing amounts of emphysema in COPD reduces the yield of BALF and therefore

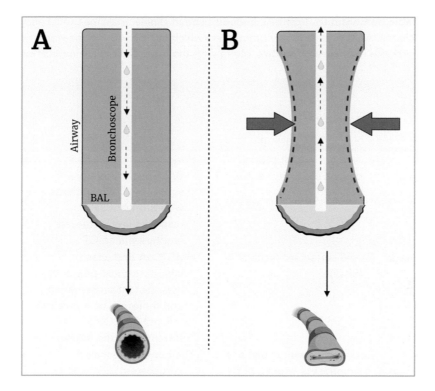

Figure 8.2 Bronchial wall collapse under negative pressure. Upon insertion of a bronchoscope and saline, the airways remain dilated (A). Subsequent removal of lavage creates negative pressure within the airways and can lead to bronchial wall collapse (B). BAL: bronchoalveolar lavage.

the efficacy of alveolar sampling (8). They used a validated emphysema index to quantify the significance of emphysema, which correlates with reduced BALF yield. One such explanation for the reduced yield was an increase in compliance of the bronchial walls, which collapse on negative pressure (suction) via the bronchoscope leading to less return of fluid. This concept is demonstrated in Figure 8.2.

BAL IN COPD RESEARCH

Biomarkers are an area of research for which BAL is used extensively in COPD. Some key insights into pathophysiology and treatment revealed by BAL studies are shown in Table 8.2.

Given the invasive nature of obtaining BALF, researchers often implement alternative, less invasive sampling methods such as sputum induction. Reproducibility is of particular importance in longitudinal studies, where it may not be

appropriate to subject patients to repeat bronchoscopies. Moreover, bronchoscopy is less likely to be tolerated by patients with unstable or exacerbated disease, which limits study mainly to the stable state.

Multiple papers have shown equal efficacy of less invasive procedures for the procurement of biomarkers found in BAL (9, 10). For example, Yigla et al. demonstrated that measurements of oxidants in saliva and BALF were comparable, which is clearly less invasive, while Diken et al. showed that cotinine levels in smokers in patients with COPD are similar in serum as they are in BAL (9, 10). However, in their comparison of potential COPD biomarkers, Röpcke et al. demonstrate a poor correlation between serum and BALF biomarkers, suggesting systemic inflammation in COPD is not a spill-over from the lungs (7). This is important as it promotes the need to continue to look for biomarkers at a local alveolar level going forward, as there may

Table 8.2 The table demonstrates how BAL findings used in clinical trials for COPD and alpha-1 antitrypsin deficiency (AATD) may identify biomarkers which can be used to measure treatment effect in both clinical practice and research studies, along with the potential clinical implications of these findings

Element of pathophysiology or treatment studied	BAL findings	Potential/future clinical implications	Paper
Bronchodilator response in the presence of emphysema	Raised eosinophil cationic protein (ECP) and eotaxin-1 in BALF	Eosinophil biomarkers in BALF might identify a subset of COPD patients with bronchodilator response and increased emphysema on CT	Miller et al. (32)
Effect of simvastatin in COPD	Raised surfactant protein D (SP-D)	HMG-CoA Reductase inhibitors could play a role in surfactant preservation and therefore be a possible adjunct for COPD treatment in the future	Patyk et al. (33)
Effect of inhaled corticosteroids in COPD	Reduction in neutrophil and lymphocyte counts, but increase in macrophage counts in BALF	The benefit of inhaled corticosteroids is well established in COPD to reduce inflammatory response, which presents as recurrent infections or features of reversibility	Jen et al. (34)
	Reduction in IL-8 and neutrophils following treatment with inhaled budesonide		Ozol et al. (35)
	Reduction in PGE2, 6kPGF1alpha and PGF2alpha after treatment with inhaled fluticasone		Verhoeven et al. (36)
	Increase in SP-D expression in BALF	SP-D as also shown in the row above could become a biomarker in measures of inflammation and treatment response in COPD	Sims et al. (37)
Effect of combined LABA/ICS in COPD	Increase in the levels of pro-surfactant protein-B (pro-SFTPB) in BALF after treatment with budesonide/formoterol	Reduced levels of pro-SFTPB shown to correlate with severity of airflow obstruction and thereby COPD. Therefore, pro-SFTPB in BALF could provide information on disease severity and response to treatment	Um et al. (38)

(Continued)

Table 8.2 (Continued)

Element of pathophysiology or treatment studied	BAL findings	Potential/future clinical implications	Paper
Augmentation therapy for alpha-1 antitrypsin deficiency (AATD)	Increased levels of AAT levels in BALF following aerosolized recombinant AAT	BALF is able to demonstrate the success of augmentation therapy in AATD	Hubbard et al. (39)
	Increased levels of AAT levels in BALF following intravenous administration of AAT concentrate from pooled human plasma	This demonstrates the ability of intravenous augmentation therapy to produce higher levels of AAT in the alveolar space	Gadek et al. (40)
	Reduced desmosine and isodesmosine (DI) in BALF post augmentation therapy	Reduction in DI represents a reduction in elastin degradation in AATD and therefore can potentially be used as a biomarker for augmentation treatment effect going forward	Ma et al. (41)

still be a biomarker only available by BAL which remains undiscovered. Röpcke et al. also, however, demonstrated a correlation in concentrations of biomarkers (namely albumin (HSA), matrix metalloprotease 9 (MMP9), and MMP9/TIMP1 ratio in smoking COPD patients) between two lung compartments (BAL and induced sputum) suggesting a less invasive method of sampling may be appropriate for ascertaining airway inflammation. Conversely, an early study compared the use of induced sputum and BAL for differential cell count and cytokine concentration, which showed that differential cell counts between induced sputum and BAL were not comparable and did not correlate. The authors attributed this finding to the derivation of sample types from differing lung compartments. By contrast, the concentration of interleukin-8 (IL-8) and eosinophil cationic protein (ECP) did correlate between the two sample types (11). Researchers must therefore consider the biomarker of interest when designing studies and deciding on sample collection methods.

The use of BAL remains an important research tool, but given the availability of biomarkers in less invasive techniques such as induced sputum, it is unlikely to become more than a research tool

at present. This is, of course, unless a unique biomarker only available in BALF is found.

FUTURE USE OF BAL IN COPD

There is extensive research currently ongoing in the investigation of the alveolar environment in COPD. There is the belief that the microbiome of the alveolar environment and cytokine analysis can be useful in a variety of situations ranging from diagnosis of COPD, detecting early progression before clinical manifestation, differentiation between asthma and COPD, and identifying targets for potential therapies in the future (12–25). BAL is currently being used as the investigation of choice for research purposes looking at the small airways environment. Some examples of these are shown below.

BAL has facilitated numerous findings of the lower airway microbiome in respiratory disease. Pharyngeal contamination, present in sputum sampling methods, is of particular concern in microbiome studies because of the relatively higher bacterial burden and different composition in the upper respiratory tract. Although yet to be shown in COPD, in idiopathic pulmonary fibrosis, the study of BAL microbiota has displayed predictive potential for disease outcome (26, 27).

Proboszcz et al. have shown that interleukin-6 and interleukin-13 (IL-6/IL-13) in BALF can differentiate between asthma and COPD in their stable states (13). Although this has an impact on the treatments of choice, if there is an element of crossover between the two conditions, the phenotype demonstrates which treatments the patient should be on. For example, if there is evidence of inflammatory response demonstrated by reversibility, atopy, eosinophilia, or repeated infections, then inhaled corticosteroids are indicated, which again are also the treatment of choice for asthmatics. At present, the phenotype, along with other metrics such as lung function, which are less invasive than BAL, are adequate in diagnosing COPD and/or differentiating from asthma.

IL-6 has also shown to be elevated in the BALF of patients with COPD who have invasive pulmonary aspergillosis (IPA) (14). Fortún et al., Zhang et al., and He et al. have also looked at the role of galactomannan in BALF in the diagnosis of IPA in both hematological and critically unwell COPD patients (28–30). However, the technique for BAL varied in these papers with He et al. only using 60 ml of infiltrated fluid, rather than the standard 150 ml, which could raise the question of whether we class this as a true BAL or a bronchial washing. The sensitivity point also varied with He et al. quoting 0.8 and Zhang et al. quoting 1.25 as a cut-off for the galactomannan level in diagnosing IPA. This finding in conjunction with serum galactomannan could help to diagnose IPA. However, the sensitivity and specificity of these findings in BALF is comparable to the specificity and sensitivity of serum analysis, which as mentioned before, is a less invasive test and therefore currently preferable if this was to be used in clinical practice.

One area showing promising research is micro-RNA (miRNA), which has been shown to be a potential biomarker for COPD and other inflammatory airway diseases (15). It has been shown to increase the chance of diagnosing COPD prior to clinical manifestation and may well be an area of future clinical use of BAL. In addition to this, Couëtil et al. demonstrated that BAL cytology can show early detection of inflammatory respiratory diseases in horses (21). Although these were not specific to COPD, it gives further evidence to the need for further research into the use of BAL for diagnosis.

BALF differential cell count has been shown to demonstrate the different phenotypes of COPD found clinically (31). However, these again may be detectable clinically without the need for invasive testing. For example, increased eosinophils in the BALF may show patients who would be responsive to steroids, but the features of inflammation found clinically would already predict this.

CONCLUSION

BAL is a procedure which is used often for COPD research. As of now, there is no viable indication for the use of BAL in the clinical management or investigation of COPD. There is clear evidence that increasing amounts of emphysema in patients with COPD reduces the yield found from BALF, which makes it less reliable as an investigation. As such, the selection of patients for both research and clinical reasons for BAL is important. Optimization of the underlying COPD and careful management of sedation within the procedure increases the safety of BAL in COPD patients. There is an increased risk of complications with COPD patients, but the research does not seem to show that these are long-lasting. Much work is ongoing in the use of BAL to identify biomarkers, cytokines, and the microbiome in the alveolar bed, which may be used to identify future therapies in the management of COPD. However, there is also good evidence that other methods of collecting samples, such as induced sputum and serum, are just as sensitive/specific. So, even though BALF may identify biomarkers that can be used going forward, other less invasive sampling techniques may yield similar results and are therefore more likely to be used in clinical practice. BAL continues to be a useful tool for research in COPD going forward.

REFERENCES

1. Global Initiative for Chronic Obstructive Lung Disease. Global strategy for the diagnosis, management, and prevention of chronic obstructive pulmonary disease 2022 report. https://goldcopd.org/2022-gold-reports-2/.

2. Du Rand IA, Blaikley J, Booton R, Chaudhuri N, Gupta V, Khalid S, et al. British Thoracic Society guideline for diagnostic flexible bronchoscopy in adults: Accredited by NICE. *Thorax.* 2013;68(Suppl 1):i1.

3. Leiten EO, Eagan TML, Martinsen EMH, Nordeide E, Husebø GR, Knudsen KS, et al. Complications and discomfort after research bronchoscopy in the MicroCOPD study. *BMJ Open Respiratory Research.* 2020;7(1):e000449.

4. Wells JM, Arenberg DA, Barjaktarevic I, Bhatt SP, Bowler RP, Christenson SA, et al. Safety and tolerability of comprehensive research bronchoscopy in chronic obstructive pulmonary disease. Results from the SPIROMICS bronchoscopy substudy. *Annals of the American Thoracic Society.* 2019;16(4):439–46.

5. Hattotuwa K, Gamble EA, O'Shaughnessy T, Jeffery PK, Barnes NC. Safety of bronchoscopy, biopsy, and BAL in research patients with COPD. *Chest.* 2002;122(6):1909–12.

6. Bellinger CR, Khan I, Chatterjee AB, Haponik EF. Bronchoscopy safety in patients with chronic obstructive lung disease. *Journal of Bronchology and Interventional Pulmonology.* 2017;24(2):98–103.

7. Röpcke S, Holz O, Lauer G, Müller M, Rittinghausen S, Ernst P, et al. Repeatability of and relationship between potential COPD biomarkers in bronchoalveolar lavage, bronchial biopsies, serum, and induced sputum. *PLOS ONE.* 2012;7(10):e46207.

8. Löfdahl JM, Cederlund K, Nathell L, Eklund A, Sköld CM. Bronchoalveolar lavage in COPD: Fluid recovery correlates with the degree of emphysema. *European Respiratory Journal.* 2005;25(2):275.

9. Yigla M, Berkovich Y, Nagler RM. Oxidative stress indices in COPD—Broncho-alveolar lavage and salivary analysis. *Archives of Oral Biology.* 2007;52(1):36–43.

10. Diken OE, Unculu S, Karnak D, Cağlayan O, Göçmen JS, Kayacan O. Cotinine levels in serum and bronchoalveolar lavage fluid. *Southeast Asian Journal of Tropical Medicine and Public Health.* 2010;41(5):1252–7.

11. Rutgers SR, Timens W, Kaufmann HF, van der Mark TW, Koeter GH, Postma DS. Comparison of induced sputum with bronchial wash, bronchoalveolar lavage and bronchial biopsies in COPD. *European Respiratory Journal.* 2000;15(1):109.

12. Pelaia G, Terracciano R, Vatrella A, Gallelli L, Busceti MT, Calabrese C, et al. Application of proteomics and peptidomics to COPD. *BioMed Research International.* 2014;2014:764581.

13. Proboszcz M, Paplińska-Goryca M, Nejman-Gryz P, Górska K, Krenke R. A comparative study of sTREM-1, IL-6 and IL-13 concentration in bronchoalveolar lavage fluid in asthma and COPD: A preliminary study. *Advances in Clinical and Experimental Medicine: Official Organ Wroclaw Medical University.* 2017;26(2):231–6.

14. Liu F, Zhang X, Du W, Du J, Chi Y, Sun B, et al. Diagnosis values of IL-6 and IL-8 levels in serum and bronchoalveolar lavage fluid for invasive pulmonary aspergillosis in chronic obstructive pulmonary disease. *Journal of Investigative Medicine: The Official Publication of the American Federation for Clinical Research.* 2021;69(7):1344.

15. Kaur G, Maremanda KP, Campos M, Chand HS, Li F, Hirani N, et al. Distinct exosomal miRNA profiles from BALF and lung tissue of COPD and IPF patients. *International Journal of Molecular Sciences.* 2021;22(21):11830.

16. Lozo Vukovac E, Miše K, Gudelj I, Perić I, Duplančić D, Vuković I, et al. Bronchoalveolar pH and inflammatory biomarkers in patients with acute exacerbation of chronic obstructive pulmonary disease. *The Journal of International Medical Research.* 2019;47(2):791–802.

17. Wendt CH, Nelsestuen G, Harvey S, Gulcev M, Stone M, Reilly C. Peptides in bronchoalveolar lavage in chronic obstructive pulmonary disease. *PLOS ONE*. 2016;11(5):e0155724.

18. Pattarayan D, Thimmulappa RK, Ravikumar V, Rajasekaran S. Diagnostic potential of extracellular microRNA in respiratory diseases. *Clinical Reviews in Allergy and Immunology*. 2018;54(3):480–92.

19. Hollander C, Sitkauskiene B, Sakalauskas R, Westin U, Janciauskiene SM. Serum and bronchial lavage fluid concentrations of IL-8, SLPI, sCD14 and sICAM-1 in patients with COPD and asthma. *Respiratory Medicine*. 2007;101(9):1947–53.

20. Gupta S, Shariff M, Chaturvedi G, Sharma A, Goel N, Yadav M, et al. Comparative analysis of the alveolar microbiome in COPD, ECOPD, sarcoidosis, and ILD patients to identify respiratory illnesses specific microbial signatures. *Scientific Reports*. 2021;11(1):3963.

21. Couëtil LL, Rosenthal FS, DeNicola DB, Chilcoat CD. Clinical signs, evaluation of bronchoalveolar lavage fluid, and assessment of pulmonary function in horses with inflammatory respiratory disease. *American Journal of Veterinary Research*. 2001;62(4):538–46.

22. Tzortzaki EG, Tsoumakidou M, Makris D, Siafakas NM. Laboratory markers for COPD in "susceptible" smokers. *Clinica Chimica Acta*. 2006;364(1):124–38.

23. Soni S, Garner JL, O'Dea KP, Koh M, Finney L, Tirlapur N, et al. Intra-alveolar neutrophil-derived microvesicles are associated with disease severity in COPD. *American Journal of Physiology-Lung Cellular and Molecular Physiology*. 2020;320(1):L73–L83.

24. Gorska K, Krenke R, Domagala-Kulawik J, Korczynski P, Nejman-Gryz P, Kosciuch J, et al. Comparison of cellular and biochemical markers of airway inflammation in patients with mild-to-moderate asthma and chronic obstructive pulmonary disease: An induced sputum and bronchoalveolar lavage fluid study. *Journal of Physiology and Pharmacology : An Official Journal of the Polish Physiological Society*. 2008;59(Suppl 6):271–83.

25. Casado B, Iadarola P, Luisetti M, Kussmann M. Proteomics-based diagnosis of chronic obstructive pulmonary disease: The hunt for new markers. *Expert Review of Proteomics*. 2008;5(5):693–704.

26. Molyneaux PL, Cox MJ, Willis-Owen SAG, Mallia P, Russell KE, Russell A-M, et al. The role of bacteria in the pathogenesis and progression of idiopathic pulmonary fibrosis. *American Journal of Respiratory and Critical Care Medicine*. 2014;190(8):906–13.

27. Han MK, Zhou Y, Murray S, Tayob N, Noth I, Lama VN, et al. Lung microbiome and disease progression in idiopathic pulmonary fibrosis: An analysis of the COMET study. *The Lancet Respiratory Medicine*. 2014;2(7):548–56.

28. Fortún J, Martín-Dávila P, Gomez Garcia de la Pedrosa E, Silva JT, Garcia-Rodríguez J, Benito D, et al. Galactomannan in bronchoalveolar lavage fluid for diagnosis of invasive aspergillosis in non-hematological patients. *Journal of Infection*. 2016;72(6):738–44.

29. Zhang X-B, Chen G-P, Lin Q-C, Lin X, Zhang H-Y, Wang J-H. Bronchoalveolar lavage fluid galactomannan detection for diagnosis of invasive pulmonary aspergillosis in chronic obstructive pulmonary disease. *Medical Mycology*. 2013;51(7):688–95.

30. He H, Ding L, Sun B, Li F, Zhan Q. Role of galactomannan determinations in bronchoalveolar lavage fluid samples from critically ill patients with chronic obstructive pulmonary disease for the diagnosis of invasive pulmonary aspergillosis: A prospective study. *Critical Care*. 2012;16(4):R138.

31. Shimura S. [Bronchoalveolar lavage in diagnosis of chronic obstructive pulmonary disease]. *Nihon Rinsho Japanese Journal of Clinical Medicine*. 1999;57(9):2005–11.

32. Miller M, Ramsdell J, Friedman PJ, Cho JY, Renvall M, Broide DH. Computed tomographic scan–diagnosed chronic obstructive pulmonary disease–emphysema: Eotaxin-1 is associated with bronchodilator response and extent of emphysema. *Journal of Allergy and Clinical Immunology*. 2007;120(5):1118–25.

33. Patyk I, Rybacki C, Kalicka A, Rzeszotarska A, Korsak J, Chciałowski A. Simvastatin therapy and bronchoalveolar lavage fluid biomarkers in chronic obstructive pulmonary disease. In: Pokorski M, editor. *Pulmonary Health and Disorders*. Cham: Springer International Publishing; 2019, pp. 43–52.

34. Jen R, Rennard SI, Sin DD. Effects of inhaled corticosteroids on airway inflammation in chronic obstructive pulmonary disease: A systematic review and meta-analysis. *International Journal of Chronic Obstructive Pulmonary Disease*. 2012;7:587–95.

35. Ozol D, Aysan T, Solak ZA, Mogulkoc N, Veral A, Sebik F. The effect of inhaled corticosteroids on bronchoalveolar lavage cells and IL-8 levels in stable COPD patients. *Respiratory Medicine*. 2005;99(12):1494–500.

36. Verhoeven GT, Garrelds IM, Hoogsteden HC, Zijlstra FJ. Effects of fluticasone propionate inhalation on levels of arachidonic acid metabolites in patients with chronic obstructive pulmonary disease. *Mediators of Inflammation*. 2001;10(1):692172.

37. Sims MW, Tal-Singer RM, Kierstein S, Musani AI, Beers MF, Panettieri RA, et al. Chronic obstructive pulmonary disease and inhaled steroids alter surfactant protein D (SP-D) levels: A cross-sectional study. *Respiratory Research*. 2008;9(1):13.

38. Um SJ, Lam S, Coxson H, Man SFP, Sin DD. Budesonide/formoterol enhances the expression of pro surfactant protein-B in lungs of COPD patients. *PLOS ONE*. 2013;8(12):e83881.

39. Hubbard RC, McElvaney NG, Sellers SE, Healy JT, Czerski DB, Crystal RG. Recombinant DNA-produced alpha 1-antitrypsin administered by aerosol augments lower respiratory tract antineutrophil elastase defenses in individuals with alpha 1-antitrypsin deficiency. *The Journal of Clinical Investigation*. 1989;84(4):1349–54.

40. Gadek JE, Klein HG, Holland PV, Crystal RG. Replacement therapy of alpha 1-antitrypsin deficiency. Reversal of protease-antiprotease imbalance within the alveolar structures of PiZ subjects. *The Journal of Clinical Investigation*. 1981;68(5):1158–65.

41. Ma S, Lin YY, He J, Rouhani FN, Brantly M, Turino GM. Alpha-1 antitrypsin augmentation therapy and biomarkers of elastin degradation. *COPD: Journal of Chronic Obstructive Pulmonary Disease*. 2013;10(4):473–81.

9

Cystic fibrosis and non-CF bronchiectasis: Cystic Fibrosis

FLORIAN STEHLING

INTRODUCTION

Cystic fibrosis (CF) is a monogenetic disorder caused by mutations in the cystic fibrosis transmembrane conductance regulator (CFTR) gene (Shteinberg et al., 2021). CFTR dysfunction results in disturbed epithelial ion transport for chloride, sodium, and bicarbonate. The consequence of the disturbed ion flow is the emergence of viscous secretions, mainly in the lungs predisposing to chronic infection and neutrophilic airway inflammation, which results in progressive lung damage. The primary locations of bacterial (fungal) bronchitis are the peripheral airways resulting in small airway disease. In the further course of the disease a vicious cycle of mucus plugging, neutrophilic inflammation, and infection leads to destruction of the airway and lung tissue and additionally affects medium-sized airways where bronchiectasis develops. The lung parenchyma undergoes atelectasis, collapse, and pneumonia. Furthermore, the persistent inflammation may cause dilatation and neovascularization of the bronchial arteries often leading to hemoptysis.

Systematic evaluation of early CF lung disease during the Australian early surveillance program AREST-CF showed that neutrophilic inflammation and bacterial colonization are frequently already observed in infants and progresses by age. Free neutrophil elastase activity in the airways (detected in the BAL) contributes to lung damage and predicts the development of persistent bronchiectasis (Sly et al., 2013). Airway colonization of CF patients is age dependent with the CF-characteristic Gram-negative rods becoming more prevalent during adolescence. Over the course of a life with CF a complex microbiome of a variety of bacteria and fungi establishes (Blanchard and Waters, 2019). Importantly colonization with different bacteria has different effects on the course of CF lung disease. In particular, *Pseudomonas aeruginosa* and *Mycobacterium abscessus* are known to worsen the course of lung function and survival (Qvist et al., 2016). Therefore, aggressive therapeutic strategies are recommended to eradicate certain bacteria after first isolation (e.g., for *Pseudomonas aeruginosa*). As early

DOI: 10.1201/9781003146834-11

identification of those pathogens is crucial, surveillance of the infection/colonization of the airways/lungs is a hallmark of CF care (Castellani et al., 2018).

Bronchoalveolar lavage (BAL) remains the gold standard for the diagnosis of lower airway infection. However, regular BAL as an invasive procedure is barely feasible in a large cohort of patients with CF. Surveillance is performed at least every three months by microbiologic examination of sputum samples that have a high sensitivity of 91% compared to the gold standard BAL (Jung et al., 2002). But, in non-sputum-expectorating children, alternatively employed deep throat swabs exhibit a notably lower sensitivity for the growth of *Pseudomonas aeruginosa* with 44% compared to BAL sampling (Rosenfeld et al., 1999). However, induced sputum following a structured protocol (Table 9.1) is able to detect pathogens as sensitive as the gold standard two-lobe BAL even in non-sputum-producing children (Forton, 2019).

It should be noted that routine BAL surveillance in children with CF does not improve the overall disease course in terms of lung function or *Pseudomonas aeruginosa* infection compared to oropharyngeal cultures obtained by deep cough swab (Wainwright et al., 2011). Therefore bronchoscopy-guided antimicrobial therapy for CF is not recommended (Jain et al., 2018). However, there are some established indications for bronchoscopy and BAL in CF:

Table 9.1 Structured sputum induction (Forton, 2019)

- Inhalation of hypertonic sodium chloride using a jet nebulizer
- Physiotherapy is given during and after the nebulization
- Physiotherapy may be supported by percussion, vibration, positive expiratory pressure breathing
- Oropharyngeal suction is used in patients who cannot expectorate spontaneously

Indications for bronchoscopy in CF

1. Inflammation
   Lung inflammation diagnosed in BAL is thought to contribute to the progress of lung damage in CF. Measurement of lung inflammation parameters in BAL studies has provided important insights into the pathogenesis of early CF lung disease. Elevated inflammatory parameters precede other conventional biomarkers such as spirometry and may predict the development of structural lung disease such as bronchiectasis in the asymptomatic infant (Sly et al., 2013). The main inflammatory parameters from BAL studies are polymorphonuclear (PMN) neutrophils, neutrophil elastase (NE), IL-6, and IL-8 that reflect endobronchial inflammation. IL-8 is the chemoattractant for neutrophils, the neutrophils are the effectors, and the released NE degrades lung tissue (Fayon et al., 2014). In advanced CF lung disease inflammation increases. At least in stable young adults, inflammation is more pronounced in the upper compared to the lower lobes (Meyer and Sharma, 1997). However, to date, routine monitoring of lung inflammation in BAL has no role in the routine care of CF patients.

2. Microbiology
   Bronchoscopy and BAL can help answer special microbiologic questions:
   - In general, escalation of microbiologic work-up to bronchoscopy and BAL is reserved for patients with CF who do not respond to oropharyngeal culture-directed or empirical antibiotic therapy. In this setting BAL is able to identify additional and potential causative pathogens and thus alter the management of difficult-to-treat pulmonary exacerbations (Gileles-Hillel et al., 2022).
   - Searching for a colonization/infection caused by *Pseudomonas aeruginosa*. If routine surveillance of oropharyngeal cultures remains negative, but the serologic response to *Pseudomonas aeruginosa* is present (positive antibodies against *Pseudomonas aeruginosa*) there is

a high suspicion of *Pseudomonas aeruginosa* colonization of the respiratory tract. *Pseudomonas* antibodies sometimes become positive before surveillance airway cultures (e.g., throat swabs) show *Pseudomonas* colonies (West et al., 2002). In these situations, BAL can help to detect *Pseudomonas aeruginosa* and initiate eradication therapy in a timely manner.

- Non-tuberculous mycobacteria pulmonary disease (NTM-PD) and in particular the rapidly growing *Mycobacterium abscessus* complex (MABSC) may cause significant and difficult-to-treat lung infection in CF patients. Recently published consensus recommendations for the management of NTM by the US Cystic Fibrosis Foundation and the European Cystic Fibrosis Foundation (Floto et al., 2016) underline the importance of NTM-PD in CF. When NTM-PD is suspected (worsening of respiratory symptoms, night sweats, weight loss, or fevers) work-up with a high-resolution chest computed tomography (HRCT) scan of the chest is recommended. HRCT changes suggestive of NTM-PD (inflammatory nodules, new tree-in-bud, ground glass, or cavitation) exhibit a significant overlap with CF lung disease (Figure 9.1). However, under suspicion of NTM-PD a stepwise microbiologic evaluation is warranted, starting with an examination of three expectorated or induced sputum samples. If the results of sputum testing are negative and imaging suggests NTM-PD, BAL of the most affected lung lobe is indicated. One NTM-positive BAL or two positive sputum cultures are rated diagnostic for NTM-PD in CF (Floto et al., 2016).

3. Atelectasis

Mucus plugging and lobar atelectasis are a complication of pulmonary exacerbations in CF. The development of atelectasis may be due to various factors such as general disease progression, allergic bronchopulmonary aspergillosis (ABPA), or other factors that alter the viscosity of airway secretions. No guidelines for the management of atelectasis in CF are published. The initial approach includes treatment with antibiotics combined with intensified secretolytic inhalation therapy (hypertonic saline/DNAse) and chest physiotherapy. If this strategy fails, bronchoscopy helps to assess the cause of persistent atelectasis including airway abnormalities (such as

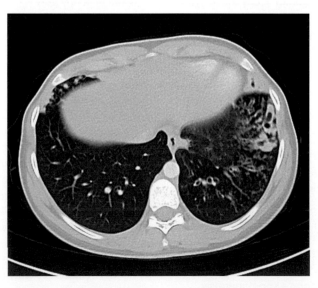

Figure 9.1 CF lung disease with classical large bronchiectasis and additional discrete tree-in-bud pattern and peripheral nodules in a CF patient without NTM-PD.

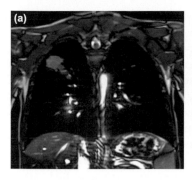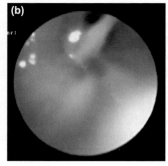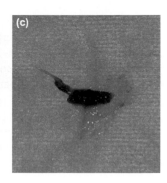

Figure 9.2 a) Localized round mass in a 9 y/o CF patient with normal lung function tests and without infectious deterioration, b) bonchoscopic view on localized mucus plugging, c) removed mucus plug.

airway malacia, which is more prevalent in CF) or casts. In addition, bronchoscopy may help to reopen the lung segment by removal of the occluding plug (Figure 9.2 (a)–(c)). The dispersion of the mucus plugging might be supported by the local (bronchoscopic) installation of DNAse (Daccò et al., 2022). All procedures must be performed in a timely manner, as persistent atelectasis may lead to irreversible lung damage with persistent shunting.

Procedure

Bronchoscopy and BAL are standard procedures, however there are published guidelines on how to perform flexible airway endoscopy in adults by the British Thoracic Society (BTS) (Du Rand et al., 2013) and in children by the European Respiratory Society (ERS) (Midulla et al., 2003). Bronchoscopy and BAL are done under deep sedation or general anesthesia. The level of sedation is determined by the overall clinical condition and the indication. In general, close cooperation between the bronchoscopist and the anesthetist is essential as they somehow compete against the airway. The examiner needs to consider the patient's comfort, the goal of the procedure, and the conditions of the bronchoscopist.

A cough swab/sputum sample must be taken on the day of the bronchoscopy to document the colonization status of the upper airways that are passed by the bronchoscope. Bronchoscopy

and BAL in CF patients may be complicated by large amounts of mucus. Additionally, persistent coughing – most likely the result of neutrophilic inflammation in CF – may complicate the procedure, even when deep sedation is combined with local anesthesia with lidocaine. When BAL procedures are performed for microbiological surveillance, several aspects need to be considered. First, local anesthesia with lidocaine applied using the spray-as-you-go technique has bactericidal effects and may contaminate the BAL fluid and therefore worsen the microbiologic culture recovery (Chandan et al., 2005). Second, a suspected infection/colonization of a certain bacteria/mold might not be uniformly distributed throughout the CF lungs (Gilchrist et al., 2011). Therefore, it is recommended to lavage at least two lobes including the middle lobe and the radiologically identified hotspot (Brennan et al., 2008; Gilchrist et al., 2011). The middle lobe is lavaged with three aliquots and the additional lobe with a single aliquot of normal saline (Brennan et al., 2008). BAL fluid is sent to microbiology for culture (including NTM, fungi), virology, and cytology for fat-laden macrophages.

Complications

Bronchoscopy and BAL are safe procedures in the hand of experienced investigators. Most adverse events are rated minor, however the majority has a transient nature like a worsening of cough occurring in up to 30% and fever during the first 24 h after BAL in up to 10% (Wainwright et al.,

2011; Gileles-Hillel et al., 2022). Serious adverse events are less frequent, but significant clinical deterioration occurs in up to 5% (Wainwright et al., 2011). At least in children, complications are more frequent than in non-CF patients (fever 30% vs 19%; severe complication 5% vs 2%) (de Blic et al., 2002; Wainwright et al., 2011), which is most likely attributed to the high number of infectious secretions in the airways of CF patients. Although antibiotic therapy for post-BAL fever is not generally recommended, the threshold in CF patients with a huge amount of putrid sputum is much lower, at least, if the bronchoscopy was performed to diagnose an unidentified respiratory infection.

In summary, bronchoscopy and BAL are rarely performed procedures in patients with CF for microbiological diagnostics in special cases or for work-up of persistent atelectasis. Especially when bronchoscopy and BAL are performed in a setting of pulmonary exacerbation, a further deterioration must be anticipated and an appropriate antibiotic regime preplanned.

NON-CF BRONCHIECTASIS

Non-CF bronchiectasis is an umbrella term for the shared final appearance of different diseases with lung involvement. The clinical syndrome of bronchiectasis includes a chronic wet cough, airway inflammation, and infection associated with abnormal bronchial dilation (Chang et al., 2021). Comparable to CF, the etiology of non-CF bronchiectasis is thought to follow an infection/inflammation paradigm that results in the destruction of bronchial and lung tissue. Neutrophilic inflammation is the key factor of bronchiectasis and results in high (uncontrolled) NE activity. The degree of neutrophilic inflammation is correlated to the bacterial load (Schäfer et al., 2018).

Indications for bronchoscopy in non-CF bronchiectasis:

- Bronchoscopy may be indicated during the differential diagnosis work-up. If sweat test, screening for primary ciliary dyskinesia, and immunological work-up do not identify a cause for bronchiectasis, further work-up

usually includes bronchoscopy and BAL to (1) exclude an airway malformation and (2) obtain microbiology including samples for mycobacterial cultures (Chang et al., 2021).

- In rare cases surgical resection of localized disease may be indicated. Bronchoscopy and BAL are indicated prior to surgery to definitely exclude foreign bodies and to obtain microbiological samples (Chang et al., 2021).

In summary, bronchoscopy and BAL are frequently performed in the initial work-up after diagnosis of non-CF bronchiectasis to provide information on the bronchial tree that might contribute to the diagnosis, but there is barely a role in routine surveillance of patients with non-CF bronchiectasis.

REFERENCES

Blanchard AC and Waters VJ (2019) Microbiology of cystic fibrosis airway disease. *Semin Respir Crit Care Med* 40(6): 727–736.

Brennan S, Gangell C, Wainwright C, et al. (2008) Disease surveillance using bronchoalveolar lavage. *Paediatr Respir Rev* 9(3): 151–159.

Castellani C, Duff AJA, Bell SC, et al. (2018) ECFS best practice guidelines: The 2018 revision. *J Cyst Fibros* 17(2): 153–178.

Chandan SS, Faoagali J and Wainwright CE (2005) Sensitivity of respiratory bacteria to lignocaine. *Pathology* 37(4): 305–307.

Chang AB, Grimwood K, Boyd J, et al. (2021) Management of children and adolescents with bronchiectasis: Summary of the ERS clinical practice guideline. *Breathe (Sheff)* 17(3): 210105.

Daccò V, Sciarrabba CS, Corti F, et al. (2022) A successful treatment of a lobar atelectasis in a patient with cystic fibrosis. *Pediatr Pulmonol* 57(11): 2868–2871.

de Blic J, Marchac V and Scheinmann P (2002) Complications of flexible bronchoscopy in children: Prospective study of 1,328 procedures. *Eur Respir J* 20(5): 1271–1276.

Du Rand IA, Blaikley J, Booton R, et al. (2013) British Thoracic Society guideline for diagnostic flexible bronchoscopy in adults: Accredited by NICE. *Thorax* 68(Suppl 1): i1–i44.

Fayon M, Kent L, Bui S, et al. (2014) Clinimetric properties of bronchoalveolar lavage inflammatory markers in cystic fibrosis. *Eur Respir J* 43(2): 610–626.

Floto RA, Olivier KN, Saiman L, et al. (2016) US cystic fibrosis foundation and European cystic fibrosis society consensus recommendations for the management of non-tuberculous mycobacteria in individuals with cystic fibrosis. *Thorax* 71(Suppl 1): i1–22.

Forton JT (2019) Detecting respiratory infection in children with cystic fibrosis: Cough swab, sputum induction or bronchoalveolar lavage. *Paediatr Respir Rev* 31: 28–31.

Gilchrist FJ, Salamat S, Clayton S, et al. (2011) Bronchoalveolar lavage in children with cystic fibrosis: How many lobes should be sampled? *Arch Dis Child* 96(3): 215–217.

Gileles-Hillel A, Yochi Harpaz L, Breuer O, et al. (2022) The clinical yield of bronchoscopy in the management of cystic fibrosis: A retrospective multicenter study. *Pediatr Pulmonol.* Epub ahead of print 20221031. DOI: 10.1002/ppul.26216.

Jain K, Wainwright C and Smyth AR (2018) Bronchoscopy-guided antimicrobial therapy for cystic fibrosis. *Cochrane Database Syst Rev* 9(9): Cd009530.

Jung A, Kleinau I, Schönian G, et al. (2002) Sequential genotyping of *Pseudomonas aeruginosa* from upper and lower airways of cystic fibrosis patients. *Eur Respir J* 20(6): 1457–1463.

Meyer KC and Sharma A (1997) Regional variability of lung inflammation in cystic fibrosis. *Am J Respir Crit Care Med* 156(5): 1536–1540.

Midulla F, de Blic J, Barbato A, et al. (2003) Flexible endoscopy of paediatric airways. *Eur Respir J* 22(4): 698–708.

Qvist T, Taylor-Robinson D, Waldmann E, et al. (2016) Comparing the harmful effects of nontuberculous mycobacteria and Gram negative bacteria on lung function in patients with cystic fibrosis. *J Cyst Fibros* 15(3): 380–385.

Rosenfeld M, Emerson J, Accurso F, et al. (1999) Diagnostic accuracy of oropharyngeal cultures in infants and young children with cystic fibrosis. *Pediatr Pulmonol* 28(5): 321–328.

Schäfer J, Griese M, Chandrasekaran R, et al. (2018) Pathogenesis, imaging and clinical characteristics of CF and non-CF bronchiectasis. *BMC Pulm Med* 18(1): 79.

Shteinberg M, Haq IJ, Polineni D, et al. (2021) Cystic fibrosis. *Lancet* 397(10290): 2195–2211.

Sly PD, Gangell CL, Chen L, et al. (2013) Risk factors for bronchiectasis in children with cystic fibrosis. *N Engl J Med* 368(21): 1963–1970.

Wainwright CE, Vidmar S, Armstrong DS, et al. (2011) Effect of bronchoalveolar lavage-directed therapy on *Pseudomonas aeruginosa* infection and structural lung injury in children with cystic fibrosis: A randomized trial. *JAMA* 306(2): 163–171.

West SE, Zeng L, Lee BL, et al. (2002) Respiratory infections with *Pseudomonas aeruginosa* in children with cystic fibrosis: Early detection by serology and assessment of risk factors. *JAMA* 287(22): 2958–2967.

10

BAL in malignancy

JOANNA DOMAGAŁA-KULAWIK

INTRODUCTION

Malignant diseases are the most serious and common entities among many chronic lung disorders. These include primary malignant neoplasms: non-small cell lung cancer (NSCLC) and small cell lung cancer (SCLC) and rare primary neoplasms. Metastases from other primary sites like breast, colon, stomach, kidney, and prostate are not insignificant. Lung cancer is placed on the top of the table of incidence and mortality from neoplasms: it kills about 2 million people annually (1). Histological diagnosis is crucial for confirmation of lung cancer. The histological diagnosis, the stage of the disease, the status of patient performance, and the status of some biomarkers are the basis for appropriate treatment and prognosis (2). Here, the precise histological and molecular diagnosis is critical. The efforts of researchers are heading to the development and improvement of diagnosis with the most accurate, relatively low-invasive techniques that bring specific and quick results. Bronchoalveolar lavage fluid (BALF) analysis is not the main method in the diagnosis of lung cancer, but it is found to be very important in this process in many aspects (3).

The "normal" constituents of BALF are immune cells and there should be nothing else. However, in different pulmonary disorders other pathological particles could be found, like microbes, epithelial cells, particles, and malignant cells. It may be an incidental finding or happen in the case of the diagnosis of peripheral lung opacities. For defined peripheral tumors, other techniques have recently been more effective than BAL. Yet, pulmonary malignancy sometimes has an image not of a solid tumor but of disseminated spread and then the role of BAL increases significantly. Such an image is typical for some forms of lung adenocarcinoma, lymphoproliferative disorders, or lymphangitic carcinomatosis. Recently, the liquid biopsy method has been developed and applied in oncology, mainly for molecular diagnosis. BAL has proven to be an effective type of liquid biopsy.

METHODOLOGICAL CONSIDERATIONS

In routine clinical practice the analysis of BALF is quantitative (4–6). The total cell count and the differential immune cell count are essential

DOI: 10.1201/9781003146834-12

and fundamental in BALF analysis. However, it should be recommended to treat this material like any biological samples obtained from humans and also perform a qualitative analysis. It makes it possible to obtain a full pattern and to find and identify "unexpected" cells. For a differential cell count the May–Grünwald–Giemsa (MGG) staining is recommended. However, the analysis of malignant features of epithelial cells in MGG is difficult and Papanicolaou, Diff-Quik, or hematoxylin-eosin staining could be suggested (it requires prior fixation of cell smears in alcohol) (7). Recently, in diagnostic cytopathology, the preparation of cell blocks from cellular materials is required (8). Cell blocks enable the preservation of material for a precise diagnosis using immunohistochemistry or other techniques, for molecular diagnosis and archiving the material. It also concerns BALF. Flow cytometry is another useful technique. BALF is a natural cell suspension and qualifies well for analysis with this technique. The spectrum of antibodies enables the recognition of the cell phenotype, the expression of molecules in or on the cells, and the concentration of cytokines (9). Flow cytometry may be perceived as an additional technique. There is a need to analyze fresh BAL samples; the spectrum of analyzed cells is rather foreseeable and planned.

Apart from the analysis of cells, the useful part of BALF is supernatant (4, 10). After centrifugation, this material can be divided into aliquots and stored frozen (−80°C) for further analyses. Subsequently, it enables the measurement of soluble factors by different techniques depending on the needs.

DIAGNOSIS OF PULMONARY MALIGNANCIES

Some examples of studies published from the early 1980s supported the value of BALF in the diagnosis of hematologic malignancies (3). Next, good results were reported for bronchioloalveolar carcinoma (BAC), at that time an often-recognized important subtype of lung adenocarcinoma. These former studies showed quite good results in the diagnosis of peripheral tumors (11–14). Some results were supported by measurement of cancer

markers, but it has not been validated to date (15). Nowadays the value of these studies is devaluing, seeing that:

- histological classifications of lung cancer as well as metastatic neoplasms have changed and are successively changing;
- much more precise histological diagnosis is required: recognition of the subtypes of NSCLC by immunohistochemistry, confirmation of molecular alterations, evaluation of the expression of PD-L1, recognition of neuroendocrine differentiation;
- for the diagnosis of peripheral lesions more accurate techniques with more effectiveness than BAL are preferable: transthoracic needle aspiration, different systems of navigation, endobronchial ultrasound techniques, or cryo-biopsy (16).

The epithelial tumor cells in the BALF smear present typical features visible in other liquid materials, like pleural and other body cavity fluids. These are three-dimensional clusters of cells. They are different in shape and size with nuclear polymorphism, hyperchromatic nuclei, and sometimes nucleoli, with a high nuclear/cytoplasmic ratio (17). However, it is sometimes difficult to recognize cell features in these clusters (Figure 10.1).

The lungs are often a location of metastases (18). The manifestation of metastases in the lungs commonly takes the form of solitary or multiple coin lesions. However, it may be presented as alveolar nodules, lymphangitic carcinomatosis, a pneumonia-like pattern, a desquamative interstitial pneumonia (DIP)-like pattern, intravascular, interstitial dissemination mimicking interstitial lung disease or alveolar hemorrhage. BAL procedure is helpful in the diagnosis of metastases (19). Lymphangitic carcinomatosis is the term for tumors spread through the lymphatics of the lung. It is a common manifestation of the spread of such aggressive tumors like adenocarcinoma of the stomach, breast, lung, prostate, pancreas, or ovary. The precise diagnosis of the origin of cancer cells needs to use additional methods, like immunocytochemistry or molecular techniques

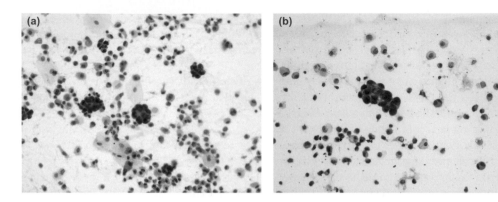

Figure 10.1 Cancer cells visible as clusters, three-dimensional groups in bronchoalveolar lavage fluid smear. (a) Hematoxylin-eosin staining. (b) May–Grünwald–Giemsa stain.

(20). Lymphangitic carcinomatosis may be the first manifestation of malignancy and in these cases, the usefulness of BAL was emphasized in clinical practice (21).

Lymphoproliferative disorders occur in the respiratory tract and may present as a spread of a generalized lymphoproliferative disease or primarily originate from bronchial associated lymphoid tissue (18). The manifestation could be the presence of diffuse lung infiltrates and it is an indication for BAL. The main cytological BALF finding is the presence of elevated lymphocytosis and sometimes the morphological features of immune cell proliferation (3). Such a finding is only informative, and the application of immunocytochemistry methods is necessary for a precise diagnosis. Flow cytometry could be a method of choice to recognize and classify hematopoietic neoplasms. Additionally, in the case of hematological disorders BAL has a wide role in a comprehensive differential diagnosis including a large spectrum of infections with the opportunistic ones and infiltration by primary proliferation (22). Thus, a full range of methods of BALF analysis should be primarily planned in patients with known or suspected lymphoproliferative disorder.

There are many secondary reactive/inflammatory changes in the lung which accompany the tumor. These are hemorrhage, thromboembolic changes, eosinophilic infiltration, organizing pneumonia, airway infections, and even sarcoidal reaction (23). The features of all of these complications could be visible in the BALF, creating associated secondary indirect abnormalities.

Bronchial epithelial cells are occasionally visible in normal BALF smears and could be confusing for an untrained eye. These cells could be changed, reactive, and even metaplastic or dysplastic. It is a normal finding in the respiratory tract, which is continuously affected by pollutants, microbes, or tobacco smoke. These cells might mimic cancer cells causing a false positive diagnosis, therefore support from an experienced pathologist would be needed. In particular, the alveolar epithelial (AE) cells are highly reactive in response to many lung pathologies: interstitial pneumonitis, diffuse alveolar damage, viral infections, lung infarction, or radiation therapy (author observations). Small clusters of AE cells may resemble the forms of adenocarcinoma. It needs special care.

To conclude, a solid tumor located in a peripheral part of the lung today is not an indication for BAL for its histological diagnosis. However, in cases of disseminated lesions of unknown origin this method could be very helpful. The main possible finding could be the presence of malignant cells (lung adenocarcinoma, lymphoma, or lymphatic spread of metastatic neoplasm). The histological examination of cell blocks is necessary for a precise diagnosis of such cells.

LUNG CANCER DIAGNOSIS AND THE EVALUATION OF PREDICTIVE BIOMARKERS

The last decade has brought important changes in the classification of malignant tumors resulting from a well-established knowledge of molecular pathways of oncogenesis. Many specialists acknowledge that alterations have become and continue to be the basis of effective treatment. Also, lung cancer therapy has recently been getting more and more individualized depending on biomarker constellation (24). The importance of these biomarkers is well-established, and their detection may serve for the diagnosis of lung cancer, its prognosis, and prediction of treatment response (25, 26). The problems with obtaining adequate cancer tissue for full evaluation in the process of diagnosis and further, in the course of treatment, led to the discovering of the value of liquid biopsy (27). A classic example of liquid biopsy is plasma, but in the case of lung cancer BALF (eventually bronchial washing, pleural fluid) was found to be superior to other plasma in many studies. It could be assumed that in the near future, the molecular pattern will serve for diagnosing a specific cancer type, thus the value of liquid biopsy with BAL will become stronger and valid.

BALF analysis may be useful in the evaluation of molecular addiction in lung cancer. A wide analysis of molecular changes by the newest methods available, e.g., multiplex platforms like Next Generation Sequencing (NGS) is recommended before treatment. It includes *EGFR* mutation status, *T790M* testing, ALK rearrangements, *ROS1* rearrangements, *BRAF* V600 mutation status, and *NTRK* rearrangements. Tests for *MET* exon 14 skipping mutations, *MET* amplifications, *RET* rearrangements, *KRAS* G12C mutations, and *HER2* mutations should be carried out (28, 29). Cell-free DNA (cfDNA) (liquid biopsy) can be used to test for oncogenic drivers (30). It was shown that the detection of cfDNA can be measured in BALF for the evaluation of the molecular status of lung cancer with high accuracy. The value of that measurement applies to situations where cancer tissue is not available. BALF, as an excellent example of liquid biopsy, could be recommended.

Other biomarkers in the BALF, like epigenetic alterations, proteins, metabolites, and microbes, were found to be of value in the diagnosis of lung cancer and in the prognosis; however, to date they have not been fully validated (30). The main directions in the studies on useful biomarkers are presented in Figure 10.2 and Figure 10.3.

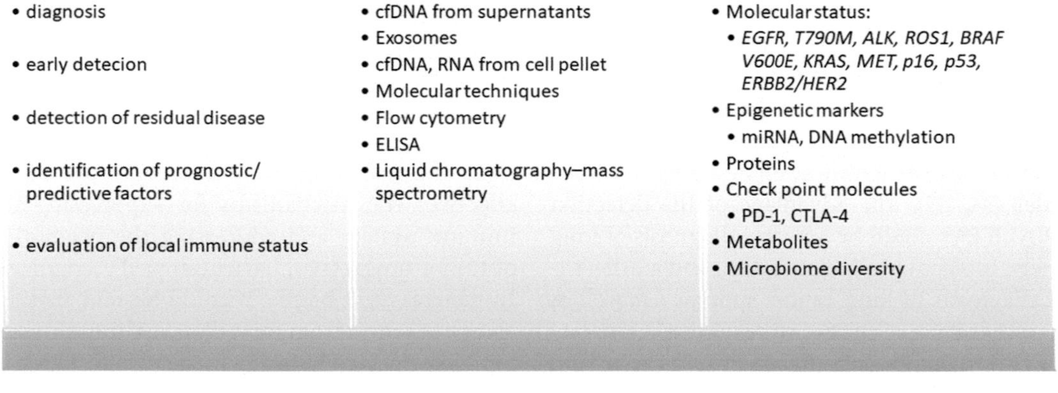

Evaluation of biomarkers for lung cancer in bronchoalveolar lavage fuid

Objective:	Methods:	Examples:
• diagnosis	• cfDNA from supernatants	• Molecular status:
	• Exosomes	• *EGFR, T790M, ALK, ROS1, BRAF*
• early detecion	• cfDNA, RNA from cell pellet	*V600E, KRAS, MET, p16, p53,*
	• Molecular techniques	*ERBB2/HER2*
• detection of residual disease	• Flow cytometry	• Epigenetic markers
	• ELISA	• miRNA, DNA methylation
• identification of prognostic/	• Liquid chromatography–mass	• Proteins
predictive factors	spectrometry	• Check point molecules
		• PD-1, CTLA-4
• evaluation of local immune status		• Metabolites
		• Microbiome diversity

Figure 10.2 Biomarkers for lung cancer possibly identified in bronchoalveolar lavage fluid for evaluation, method, and example purposes.

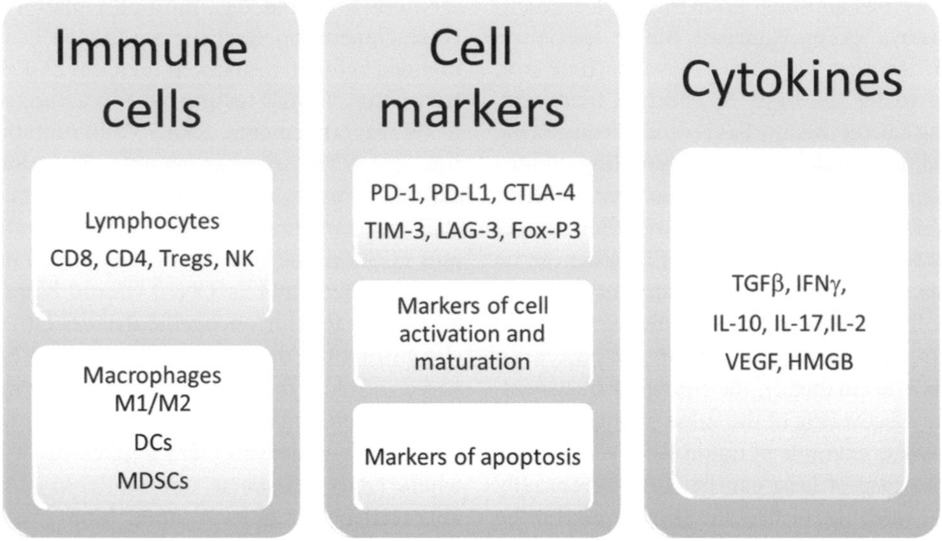

Figure 10.3 Elements of an immune reaction identified in bronchoalveolar lavage fluid of potential significance in the evaluation of the local anti-cancer response, "immunoscoring." Abbreviations: CTLA-4 – cytotoxic T lymphocyte antigen-4, DCs – dendritic cells, MDSCs – myeloid derived suppressor cells, NK – natural killer cells, NKT – natural killer T cells, PD-1 – programmed death-1, PD-L1 – programmed death-1 ligand, Tregs – regulatory T cells, TGFβ – transforming growth factor β.

Exosomes are very promising constituents of liquid biopsy. Exosomes are small extracellular vesicles (EVs) originating from different cells, i.e., from cancer cells (31, 32). They bear the antigenic and molecular cell signature with high specificity and are involved in the spread of tumors and the progression of malignant disease. It is found that exosomes are capable of the modification of the tumor environment by the strong expression of immunosuppressive molecules like programmed death-1 ligand (PD-L1), Fas-L, tumor-necrosis factor related apoptosis-inducing ligand (TRAIL), and tumor antigens (31, 33). Exosomes have been identified in BALF and the results are promising. The main barrier in research is the methodology of identification of these small molecules (34, 35). The advantage of the detection of BALF EVs could be an early diagnosis of lung cancer, molecular characteristics, and a differential diagnosis of lung cancer subtypes as well as the recognition of prognostic and predictive factors (32). A high concordance of EVs cargo with cancer tissue characteristics was found. The new direction is the use of EVs in therapy (35). It could

be achieved by the modification of their interaction with the tumor microenvironment (TME) or by the use of a natural drug delivery system.

The usefulness of the evaluation of biomarkers for lung cancer in clinical practice is not included in the guidelines. However, looking at the large number of publications it is close to application in some aspects.

BAL IN THE EVALUATION OF LOCAL IMMUNE STATUS IN LUNG CANCER

The immune status of patients with malignancy has been the center of attention for oncologists since the results of immunotherapy proved so effective. The mechanisms for suppressing the immune system and addressing the promotion of tumor progression have been well recognized. In general, very briefly, it could be said that the escape of cancer from surveillance of immune system is connected with the ineffective function of cytotoxic T cells which is carried by many mechanisms (36). One of them is the overexpression of suppressor molecules on immune cells, so-called immune checkpoints. The issue of solid tumor immunotherapy is the blockade of these checkpoints by checkpoint inhibitors (ICIs), mainly of the line PD-1–PD-L1 and CTLA-4 (37). An arena of the complicated mechanisms of anti-cancer–pro-cancer immune reactions is the TME, consisting of immune cells, mediators, and structural cells. In the case of lung cancer, the majority of TME constituents could be identified in the BALF (Figure 10.3) (38). Furthermore, it was found that the character of this immune response may play the role of a prognostic as well as a predictive factor in some tumors. The better response to ICIs was observed in "hot" (active) tumors vs "cold" (silent) ones. "Hot" tumors are defined as those with a high proportion of immune cells, an overexpression of checkpoint molecules, and an adequate cytokine network (24). The whole spectrum of immune infiltration could be evaluated in resected tumors. In particular, the models of the role of immune infiltration reported as immuno-scoring were described in colon cancer (39). In the case of lung cancer, the model cannot be applicable as the resection rate is as low as 25%. In clinical practice, only a small biopsy or cytological biopsy is used for diagnosing in a high prevalence. Thus, obtaining cancer tissue with stroma is out of accessibility. BAL can fill this gap (Table 10.1).

The usefulness of BAL in the evaluation of local immune status in lung cancer was described a long time before the widespread introduction of immuno-oncology (40–42). These studies showed the important differences of local changes when compared with systemic ones detected in peripheral blood. These studies also showed important differences between immune reactions in lung cancer when compared to healthy individuals. Then the control groups were constructed by healthy volunteers, and it was possible to document the specificity of immune response in the lung with cancer against normal circumstances.

Since then, the studies on BAL in the evaluation of immunity of lung cancer have multiplied. Alterations in the proportion of lymphocyte subtypes (high prevalence of CD8 cells), status of immune cell maturation, expression of molecules involved in the function of cells, and soluble

Table 10.1 The advantage of bronchoalveolar fluid analysis in lung cancer in the aspect of the diagnosis of cancer, prediction, and evaluation of the tumor microenvironment

BAL in lung cancer
  may be performed in all clinical stages of the diseases, also in advanced stages when full cancer tissue is not available
  is available during the diagnosis of lung cancer
  is well-standardized and reproducible
  is a repeatable procedure and enables the evaluation of the dynamics of malignant disease course and answer to the treatment
  is an example of liquid biopsy with high specificity for molecular profiling
  in immunotherapy is informative for:
    primary immune status, modulation of immune response by treatment
    is useful for the differential diagnosis of immune-related adverse events of immunotherapy

factors were observed (9, 43–51). All the known elements of the anti-cancer immune response can be identified in the BALF and it was presented by many authors (30).

Unfortunately, their results are difficult to compare and far from validation, as the groups of patients are small and heterogenic and the results are reported in different manners.

For comparative studies we and other researchers decided to apply the lung opposite to the lung with the tumor as a "healthy," control lung. Further studies proved that in some aspects both lungs form an integrated system and there were no differences between the lung affected by cancer in comparison with the opposite, "healthy" one (9, 48).

The main obstacle for studies on the immune status in lung cancer is the dynamics of immune reaction and their huge susceptibility to internal and external factors. Tobacco smoke remains the most important factor which changes the immune reaction in the respiratory tract. The measurement of the concentration of cytokines in BALF supernatants is a valuable complement to the description of local immune answer to cancer. Many studies confirmed important changes in the concentration of some cytokines known to participate in the suppressory character of lung cancer TME.

While BAL in the evaluation of immune status in lung cancer is far from standardized and incorporated in clinics, this procedure finds its usefulness in practice in diagnosing checkpoint inhibitor pneumonitis (CIP). CIP is a relatively common adverse event of the use of ICIs (immune-related adverse events, irAE) (52, 53). The autoimmune mechanisms are involved in the pathogenesis of irAE. The clinical pattern of CIP is non-specific. It may occur during immunotherapy of different tumors, not only lung cancer. BAL analysis may have an invaluable role in a differential diagnosis as a quick, low-invasive, repeatable method with high specificity (54–56).

It may help in a differential diagnosis when evaluated for:

- infectious nature of the respiratory system involvement, including opportunistic infections (mycobacteria, cytomegalovirus (CMV), galactomannan, pneumocytosis (PCP));
- tumor progression – presence of malignant cells in the BALF;
- differential cell count, lymphocyte phenotype (at least CD4 to CD8 ratio), selected cytokine concentration (53).

CONCLUDING REMARKS

BAL has been a method of examination of the respiratory tract for about 40 years, being dedicated to the diagnosis of interstitial lung diseases and infections. In lung cancer, BALF examination is helpful in the diagnosis of lung cancer and in the diagnosis of metastases to the lung by cytological methods as well as the modern techniques of molecular analysis. BALF as a valuable kind of liquid biopsy is promising in the identification of prognostic/predictive factors for lung cancer. Many studies confirmed the usefulness of BAL in the evaluation of immune status before and during immunotherapy of lung cancer including a differential diagnosis of irAE. Thus, the place of this method in the diagnosis and treatment of malignant lung tumors remains established.

REFERENCES

1. Global Burden of Disease 2019 Cancer Collaboration, Kocarnik JM, Compton K, Dean FE, Fu W, Gaw BL, et al. Cancer incidence, mortality, years of life lost, years lived with disability, and disability-adjusted life years for 29 cancer groups from 2010 to 2019: A systematic analysis for the global burden of disease study 2019. *JAMA Oncol* 2022;8(3):420–44.
2. Thai AA, Solomon BJ, Sequist LV, Gainor JF, Heist RS. Lung cancer. *Lancet* 2021;398(10299):535–54.
3. Poletti V, Poletti G, Murer B, Saragoni L, Chilosi M. Bronchoalveolar lavage in malignancy. *Semin Respir Crit Care Med* 2007;28(5):534–45.
4. Chcialowski A, Chorostowska-Wynimko J, Fal A, Pawlowicz R, Domagala-Kulawik J. [Recommendation of the polish respiratory society for bronchoalveolar lavage (BAL) sampling, processing and analysis methods]. *Pneumonol Alergol Pol* 2011;79(2):75–89.
5. Costabel U. *Atlas of Bronchoalveolar Lavage*. Chapman & Hall Medical, 1998.
6. Meyer KC, Raghu G, Baughman RP, Brown KK, Costabel U, du Bois RM, et al. An official American Thoracic Society clinical practice guideline: The clinical utility of bronchoalveolar lavage cellular analysis in interstitial lung disease. *Am J Respir Crit Care Med* 2012;185(9):1004–14.
7. Canberk S, Montezuma D, Aydin O, Demirhas MP, Denizci B, Akbas M, et al. The new guidelines of Papanicolaou Society of Cytopathology for respiratory specimens: Assessment of risk of malignancy and diagnostic yield in different cytological modalities. *Diagn Cytopathol* 2018;46(9):725–9.
8. Jain D, Nambirajan A, Borczuk A, Chen G, Minami Y, Moreira AL, et al. Immunocytochemistry for predictive biomarker testing in lung cancer cytology. *Cancer Cytopathol* 2019;127(5):325–39.
9. Osinska I, Stelmaszczyk-Emmel A, Polubiec-Kownacka M, Dziedzic D, Domagala-Kulawik J. CD4+/CD25(high)/

FoxP3+/CD127- regulatory T cells in bronchoalveolar lavage fluid of lung cancer patients. *Hum Immunol* 2016;77(10):912–5.

10. Haslam PL, Baughman RP. Report of ERS Task Force: Guidelines for measurement of acellular components and standardization of BAL. *Eur Respir J* 1999;14(2):245–8.

11. Pirozynski M. Bronchoalveolar lavage in the diagnosis of peripheral, primary lung cancer. *Chest* 1992;102(2):372–4.

12. Rennard SI, Albera C, Carratu L, Bauer W, Eckert H, Linder J, et al. Clinical guidelines and indications for bronchoalveolar lavage (BAL): Pulmonary malignancies. *Eur Respir J* 1990;3(8):956–7, 61–9.

13. Linder J, Radio SJ, Robbins RA, Ghafouri M, Rennard SI. Bronchoalveolar lavage in the cytologic diagnosis of carcinoma of the lung. *Acta Cytol* 1987;31(6):796–801.

14. Schreiber G, McCrory DC. Performance characteristics of different modalities for diagnosis of suspected lung cancer: Summary of published evidence. *Chest* 2003;123(1):115S–28S.

15. Niklinski J, Chyczewska E, Furman M, Kowal E, Laudanski J, Chyczewski L. Usefulness of a multiple biomarker assay in bronchoalveolar lavage (BAL) and serum for the diagnosis of small cell lung cancer. *Neoplasma* 1993;40(5):305–8.

16. Nicholson AG, Tsao MS, Beasley MB, Borczuk AC, Brambilla E, Cooper WA, et al. The 2021 WHO classification of lung tumors: Impact of advances since 2015. *J Thorac Oncol* 2022;17(3):362–87.

17. Koss IG. *Diagnostic Cytology and its Histopathological Bases*. Fourth ed., J.B. Lippincott Company, 1992.

18. Dail DH, Hammar SP, Colby TV. *Pulmonary Pathology Tumors*. Springer-Varlag, 1994.

19. Velez-Perez A, Abuharb B, Bammert CE, Landon G, Gan Q. Detection of non-haematolymphoid malignancies in bronchoalveolar lavages: A cancer centre's 10 year experience. *Cytopathology* 2022;33(4):449–53.

20. Bellizzi AM. An algorithmic immunohistochemical approach to define tumor type and assign site of origin. *Adv Anat Pathol* 2020;27(3):114–63.

21. Levy H, Horak DA, Lewis MI. The value of bronchial washings and bronchoalveolar lavage in the diagnosis of lymphangitic carcinomatosis. *Chest* 1988;94(5):1028–30.

22. Brownback KR, Thomas LA, Simpson SQ. Role of bronchoalveolar lavage in the diagnosis of pulmonary infiltrates in immunocompromised patients. *Curr Opin Infect Dis* 2014;27(4):322–8.

23. Bonifazi M, Renzoni EA, Lower EE. Sarcoidosis and maligancy: The chicken and the egg? *Curr Opin Pulm Med* 2021;27(5):455–62.

24. Domagala-Kulawik J. New frontiers for molecular pathology. *Front Med (Lausanne)* 2019;6:284.

25. Calabrese F, Lunardi F, Pezzuto F, Fortarezza F, Vuljan SE, Marquette C, et al. Are there new biomarkers in tissue and liquid biopsies for the early detection of non-small cell lung cancer? *J Clin Med* 2019;8(3):1–20.

26. Griesinger F, Eberhardt W, Nusch A, Reiser M, Zahn MO, Maintz C, et al. Biomarker testing in non-small cell lung cancer in routine care: Analysis of the first 3,717 patients in the German prospective, observational, nation-wide CRISP Registry (AIO-1RK-0315). *Lung Cancer* 2021;152:174–84.

27. Rolfo C, Mack P, Scagliotti GV, Aggarwal C, Arcila ME, Barlesi F, et al. Liquid biopsy for advanced NSCLC: A consensus statement from the International Association for the Study of Lung Cancer. *J Thorac Oncol* 2021;16(10):1647–62.

28. Postmus PE, Kerr KM, Oudkerk M, Senan S, Waller DA, Vansteenkiste J, et al. Early and locally advanced non-small-cell lung cancer (NSCLC): ESMO Clinical Practice Guidelines for diagnosis, treatment and follow-up. *Ann Oncol* 2017;28(Suppl 4):iv1–iv21.

29. Planchard D, Popat S, Kerr K, Novello S, Smit EF, Faivre-Finn C, et al. Metastatic non-small cell lung cancer: ESMO Clinical Practice Guidelines for diagnosis, treatment and follow-up. *Ann Oncol* 2018;29(Suppl 4):iv192–iv237.

30. Kalkanis A, Papadopoulos D, Testelmans D, Kopitopoulou A, Boeykens E, Wauters E. Bronchoalveolar lavage fluid-isolated biomarkers for the diagnostic and prognostic assessment of lung cancer. *Diagnostics (Basel)* 2022;12(12):1–27.

31. Whiteside TL. The role of tumor-derived exosomes (TEX) in shaping anti-tumor immune competence. *Cells* 2021;10(11):1–7.

32. Tinè M, Biondini D, Damin M, Semenzato U, Bazzan E, Turato G. Extracellular vesicles in lung cancer: Bystanders or main characters? *Biology* 2023;12(2):246. https://doi.org/10.3390.

33. Whiteside TL, Diergaarde B, Hong CS. Tumor-derived exosomes (TEX) and their role in immuno-oncology. *Int J Mol Sci* 2021;22(12):1–14.

34. Dlugolecka M, Szymanski J, Zareba L, Homoncik Z, Domagala-Kulawik J, Polubiec-Kownacka M, et al. Characterization of extracellular vesicles from bronchoalveolar lavage fluid and plasma of patients with lung lesions using fluorescence nanoparticle tracking analysis. *Cells* 2021;10(12):1–28.

35. Moon B, Chang S. Exosome as a delivery vehicle for cancer therapy. *Cells* 2022;11(3):1–15.

36. Xia A, Zhang Y, Xu J, Yin T, Lu XJ. T cell dysfunction in cancer immunity and immunotherapy. *Front Immunol* 2019;10:1719.

37. Reck M, Remon J, Hellmann MD. First-line immunotherapy for non-small-cell lung cancer. *J Clin Oncol* 2022;40(6):586–97.

38. Domagala-Kulawik J. The relevance of bronchoalveolar lavage fluid analysis for lung cancer patients. *Expert Rev Respir Med* 2020;14(3):329–37.

39. Galon J, Mlecnik B, Bindea G, Angell HK, Berger A, Lagorce C, et al. Towards the introduction of the 'Immunoscore' in the classification of malignant tumours. *J Pathol* 2014;232(2):199–209.

40. Domagala-Kulawik J, Guzman J, Costabel U. Immune cells in bronchoalveolar lavage in peripheral lung cancer – Analysis of 140 cases. *Respiration* 2003;70(1):43–8.

41. Domagala-Kulawik J, Hoser G, Droszcz P, Kawiak J, Droszcz W, Chazan R. T-cell subtypes in bronchoalveolar lavage fluid and in peripheral blood from patients with primary lung cancer. *Diagn Cytopathol* 2001;25(4):208–13.

42. Hoser G, Domagala-Kulawik J, Droszcz P, Droszcz W, Kawiak J. Lymphocyte subsets differences in smokers and nonsmokers with primary lung cancer: A flow cytometry analysis of bronchoalveolar lavage fluid cells. *Med Sci Monit* 2003;9(8):BR310–BR5.

43. Naumnik W, Naumnik B, Niewiarowska K, Ossolinska M, Chyczewska E. Novel cytokines: IL-27, IL-29, IL-31 and IL-33. Can they be useful in clinical practice at the time diagnosis of lung cancer? *Exp Oncol* 2012;34(4):348–53.

44. Domagala-Kulawik J, Hoser G, Safianowska A, Grubek-Jaworska H, Chazan R. Elevated TGF-beta1 concentration in bronchoalveolar lavage fluid from patients with primary lung cancer. *Arch Immunol Ther Exp (Warsz)* 2006;54(2):143–7.

45. Kwiecien I, Skirecki T, Polubiec-Kownacka M, Raniszewska A, Domagala-Kulawik J. Immunophenotype of T cells expressing programmed Death-1 and cytotoxic T cell Antigen-4 in early lung cancer: Local vs. systemic immune response. *Cancers (Basel)* 2019;11(4):1–18.

46. Naumnik W, Panek B, Ossolinska M, Naumnik B. B cell-attracting Chemokine-1 and progranulin in bronchoalveolar lavage fluid of patients with advanced non-small cell lung cancer: New prognostic factors. *Adv Exp Med Biol* 2019;1150:11–6.

47. Zikos TA, Donnenberg AD, Landreneau RJ, Luketich JD, Donnenberg VS. Lung T-cell subset composition at the time of surgical resection is a prognostic indicator in non-small cell lung cancer. *Cancer Immunol Immunother* 2011;60(6):819–27.

48. Mariniello A, Tabbo F, Indellicati D, Tesauro M, Rezmives NA, Reale ML, et al. Comparing T cell subsets in broncho-alveolar lavage (BAL) and peripheral blood in patients with advanced lung cancer. *Cells* 2022;11(20):1–17.

49. Kopinski P, Wandtke T, Dyczek A, Wedrowska E, Rozy A, Senderek T, et al. Increased levels of interleukin 27 in patients with early clinical stages of non-small cell lung cancer. *Pol Arch Intern Med* 2018;128(2):105–14.

50. Kwiecien I, Polubiec-Kownacka M, Dziedzic D, Wolosz D, Rzepecki P, Domagala-Kulawik J. CD163 and CCR7 as markers for macrophage polarization in lung cancer microenvironment. *Cent Eur J Immunol* 2019;44(4):395–402.

51. Masuhiro K, Tamiya M, Fujimoto K, Koyama S, Naito Y, Osa A, et al. Bronchoalveolar lavage fluid reveals factors contributing to the efficacy of PD-1 blockade in lung cancer. *JCI Insight* 2022;7(9):1–14.

52. Reuss JE, Suresh K, Naidoo J. Checkpoint inhibitor pneumonitis: Mechanisms, characteristics, management strategies, and beyond. *Curr Oncol Rep* 2020;22(6):56.

53. Martins F, Sykiotis GP, Maillard M, Fraga M, Ribi C, Kuntzer T, et al. New therapeutic perspectives to manage refractory immune checkpoint-related toxicities. *Lancet Oncol* 2019;20(1):e54–e64.

54. Suresh K, Naidoo J, Zhong Q, Xiong Y, Mammen J, de Flores MV, et al. The alveolar immune cell landscape is dysregulated in checkpoint inhibitor pneumonitis. *J Clin Invest* 2019;129(10):4305–15.

55. Strippoli S, Fucci L, Negri A, Putignano D, Cisternino ML, Napoli G, et al. Cellular analysis of bronchoalveolar lavage fluid to narrow differential diagnosis of checkpoint inhibitor-related pneumonitis in metastatic melanoma. *J Transl Med* 2020;18(1):473.

56. Tanaka K, Yanagihara T, Ikematsu Y, Inoue H, Ota K, Kashiwagi E, et al. Detection of identical T cell clones in peritumoral pleural effusion and pneumonitis lesions in a cancer patient during immune-checkpoint blockade. *Oncotarget* 2018;9(55):30587–93.

11

Lung transplantation and donor lung repair

NICOLAUS SCHWERK

LUNG TRANSPLANTATION AND DONOR LUNG REPAIR

Introduction

Lung transplantation (Ltx) is an established treatment option for pediatric and adult patients with severe progressing and treatment of refractory lung diseases. Although significant progress has been made in the management of critically ill patients, surgical techniques, and medical treatment before and after Ltx during the past decades, the prognosis after Ltx remains significantly worse compared to other solid organ transplantations (Chambers et al., 2021). According to the registry of the International Society for Heart and Lung Transplantation (ISHLT), the median survival post Ltx is about 6 years in adults and children (Hayes et al., 2022; Perch et al., 2022), with some significant differences between various centers (Iablonskii et al., 2022; Khan et al., 2015). The poorer prognosis compared to other solid organ transplantations is mainly due to the continuous exposure of the lungs to the surrounding environment. On the one hand, this increases the risk of infections, and on the other hand, it leads to a continuous stimulation of the immune system, which might trigger allograft rejections. Therefore, infections are primarily responsible for death during the first year after transplantation, which is mainly due to intense immunosuppression, and chronic lung allograft dysfunction (CLAD) represents the major cause of mortality thereafter (Hayes et al., 2015). There are several risk factors for the development of CLAD. These include recurrent viral or bacterial infections, chronic colonization of the lower respiratory tract by bacteria or fungi, recurrent acute cellular or humoral rejections, gastroesophageal reflux with recurrent microaspirations, and insufficient immunosuppression (Glanville et al., 2019; Verleden et al., 2019). In order to detect a graft dysfunction at an early stage, daily lung function measurements and monitoring of vital signs are mandatory. Bronchoscopy including bronchoalveolar lavage (BAL) and transbronchial biopsy is a recommended routinely used procedure to identify and manage airway complications and to detect infections, acute cellular or humoral rejections, and CLAD (Verleden et al., 2019). However,

DOI: 10.1201/9781003146834-13

the major diagnostic role of BAL after Ltx is the proof or exclusion of infections (Martinu et al., 2020). There are numerous studies searching for potential biomarkers in bronchoalveolar fluid (BALF) to predict or diagnose acute or chronic rejections (Verleden et al., 2023a). However, currently, no robust diagnostic markers are available for routine clinical use. Nevertheless, some cytological findings and biomarkers in combination with other clinical findings can be helpful for differential diagnoses in case of respiratory complaints after Ltx. Although guidelines for the performance of BAL and the interpretation of BAL findings have been published (Du Rand et al., 2013; Haslam & Baughman, 1999; Meyer et al., 2012), transplant-specific aspects have not been sufficiently discussed there. To address this problem and to assist in standardizing practices across Ltx centers by clarifying definitions and techniques and by proposing recommendations for bronchial and alveolar samplings in lung transplant recipients a consensus document, supported by the ISHLT, was recently published (Martinu et al., 2020). The indications for bronchoscopy and BAL after Ltx can be divided into two main categories, namely surveillance and diagnostic. Surveillance refers to a scheduled protocol bronchoscopy at predetermined times in clinically stable patients without evidence of graft dysfunction. Diagnostic bronchoscopy is performed in cases of suspected pathology, such as an infection or acute rejection. Although surveillance bronchoscopies are performed in most centers all over the world, the utility has not yet been proven by prospective controlled studies. For example, it has been shown that asymptomatic infections could be found in 12–40% during surveillance bronchoscopies, especially in the first 12 months after transplantation (Girgis et al., 1995; Guilinger et al., 1995; Inoue et al., 2014; Valentine et al., 2009). However, it is unclear whether the detection and treatment of asymptomatic infections after Ltx has an impact on the development of CLAD or survival. Given the low risk when performed properly and the potential benefit, performing surveillance bronchoscopies at predetermined times 1-, 3-, 6-, and 12-months post-transplant is an acceptable schedule. A diagnostic BAL is important for the diagnosis or

exclusion of infections and is therefore strongly recommended in such scenarios (Martinu et al., 2020).

MICROBIOLOGICAL AND VIROLOGICAL ANALYSES FROM BALF

As mentioned above, infections play a relevant role in the morbidity and mortality of the immunosuppressed patient, especially during the first year after Ltx (Belperio et al., 2017; Campos et al., 2008a; Campos et al., 2008b; Engelmann et al., 2009; Gottlieb et al., 2009). For this reason, a microbiological workup should always be performed in BAF. Since opportunistic and viral infections can also cause severe disease, they should also be considered. Table 11.1 provides an overview of potentially relevant pathogens, which should be addressed.

CYTOLOGICAL ANALYSIS FROM BALF

As microscopic cytology examinations are not able to differentiate between infections or rejections (Al-Za'abi et al., 2007a; Wanner et al., 2005), the validity of BAL cytology as a routine study is a matter of controversial discussion (Al-Za'abi et al., 2007b; Walts et al., 1991). However, even if there are conflicting results on the diagnostic value of cytological studies, they can be a helpful tool in addition to microbiological examinations. Special staining of cytology specimens may be a useful adjunct for the identification of difficult-to-culture organisms, such as *Norcadia* or *Mucor* species, or in cases of suspected *Pneumocystis jirovecii* infection. Furthermore, after the exclusion of an infection, a lymphocytic or neutrophilic inflammation in BAL might be suggestive of an acute rejection (Slebos et al., 2004; Tikkanen et al., 2001) or predictive for CLAD (Neurohr et al., 2009; Reynaud-Gaubert et al., 2000; Slebos et al., 2004; Tikkanen et al., 2001). A special type of chronic allograft dysfunction is the so-called azithromycin-responsive allograft dysfunction (ARAD). It has been shown that in up to 40% of patients with bronchiolitis obliterans syndrome (BOS), significant improvement and in

Table 11.1 Microbiological, virological, and mycological workup from bronchoalveolar lavage in lung transplanted patients

Group	Pathogens	Microbial analysis methods
Bacteria	Common respiratory bacteria	Quantitative bacterial cultures
	Bacterial organisms commonly identified in cystic	Specific CF bacterial cultures
	fibrosis (CF) patients	Specific CF bacterial cultures
	– *Pseudomonas aeruginosa*	PCR, mycobacterial cultures
	– *Burkholderia cepacia*	PCR, mycobacterial cultures
	Mycobacterium tuberculosis	PCR
	Atypical mycobacteria	
	Norcardia	
Fungi	*Aspergillus fumigatus*	Fungal cultures
	Candida spp.	
	Pneumocystis jirovecii	
Viruses	Influenza A + B	PCR
	Parainfluenza 1–4	
	Respiratory syncytial virus	
	Adenovirus	
	Rhinovirus	
	Human metapneumovirus	
	Respiratory syncytial virus	
	Cytomegaly virus	
	Coronaviruses	
	SARS-Cov-2	
	Herpes simplex virus	
	Epstein–Barr virus	

some cases, even normalization of lung function could be achieved by using azithromycin (Vos et al., 2012). Because initial studies described an association between responses to azithromycin and the presence of neutrophilic inflammation in the BALF (Vandermeulen et al., 2015), the term neutrophilic reversible allograft dysfunction (NRAD) was proposed (Vanaudenaerde et al., 2008). Because it was later shown that BAL neutrophilia might not be that predictive for the response to azithromycin, it was later suggested to rename this condition as ARAD (Verleden et al., 2019). Eosinophilia in the BALF can also be associated with worse survival, particularly after a diagnosis of restrictive allograft syndrome (Verleden et al., 2014). In conclusion, although no clear cutoff values for the presence or risk of developing CLAD have been established in multicenter studies, cytological examination and differentiation of inflammatory cells in BALF may provide useful information in the evaluation of

lung transplant recipients with impaired lung function. For this reason, it is recommended that all post-transplant BAL samples should include a differential cell count with or without an absolute cell count (Martinu et al., 2020).

BAL FOR RESEARCH AND POTENTIAL BIOMARKERS

As noted above, CLAD represents the leading cause of death beyond the first year after Ltx. Affected patients are also severely limited in their quality of life and therapeutic options are very limited. For this reason, many scientific studies focus on pathophysiological mechanisms in order to find new treatment options but also on the possibility of early CLAD detection or prediction by using biomarkers. CLAD is a clinical diagnosis and defined as a persistent decline ($\geq 20\%$) in forced expiratory volume in 1 s (FEV1) from the baseline. This baseline value is calculated as the mean of the best two postoperative FEV1 measurements. It is important to realize that other reasons can also cause a similar decline in FEV1, which are not considered as a manifestation of CLAD, including physiological aging, surgical factors, mechanical factors, infection, lung neoplasms, recurrence of native lung disease, and drug-induced toxicity among others (Verleden et al., 2023b). Therefore, the requirements for biomarkers to robustly discriminate between the different causes of pulmonary function decline after Ltx are very complex, which is currently the reason why they are not yet available for routine clinical use. Since a description of all studies performed to date is beyond the scope of this chapter, Table 11.2 provides, based on a review

Table 11.2 Overview of examined biomarkers with their purpose and detected associations adapted from (Verleden et al., 2023a)

Type of allograft dysfunction	Purpose	Marker	Association	References
CLAD	Risk factor + diagnostic	Donor-derived cell-free DNA	Increased	(Bazemore et al., 2021; Schneck et al., 2022; Yang et al., 2019)
CLAD/RAS	Risk factor	Mesenchymal colony forming units	Increased	(Badri et al., 2011; Combs et al., 2020)
RAS	Risk factor + prognostic	Eosinophils	Increased	(Verleden et al., 2014; Verleden et al., 2016)
CLAD	Diagnostic	NK cells	Decreased	(Greenland et al., 2014; Verleden et al., 2014)
CLAD	Risk factor	Molecular signature of immune response	Increased	(Iasella et al., 2021; Verleden et al., 2014; Weigt et al., 2017)
CLAD	Risk factor + diagnostic + prognostic	IL6/IL-6 receptor	Increased	(Verleden et al., 2015; Wheeler et al., 2021)
RAS	Diagnostic + prognostic	M65 (epithelial cell apoptosis and cell death)	Increased	(Levy et al., 2019)
RAS	Diagnostic	Alveolar alarmins	Increased	(Saito et al., 2014)
CLAD	Risk factor	C-X-C motif chemokine receptor 3	Increased	(Shino et al., 2018; Shino et al., 2013; Shino et al., 2017)
CLAD	Risk factor	Renin-angiotensin system	Increased	(Berra et al., 2021)
RAS	Diagnostic	Humoral immunity	Increased	(Vandermeulen et al., 2016; Vandermeulen et al., 2017)
CLAD	Risk factor + prognostic	Bile acids	Increased	(Urso et al., 2021)
CLAD	Risk factor + diagnostic + prognostic	Disbalance of the microbiota	Increased	(Banday et al., 2021; Bernasconi et al., 2016; Combs et al., 2021; Das et al., 2021; Watzenboeck et al., 2022)

by Verleden et al. (2023a), an overview of cellular and soluble biomarkers that have been investigated to determine their predictive value for the presence or development of allograft dysfunction.

REFERENCES

Al-Za'abi, A. M., MacDonald, S., Geddie, W., & Boerner, S. L. (2007a). Cytologic examination of bronchoalveolar lavage fluid from immunosuppressed patients. *Diagnostic Cytopathology*, *35*(11), 710–714. doi:10.1002/dc.20741

Badri, L., Murray, S., Liu, L. X., Walker, N. M., Flint, A., Wadhwa, A., & Lama, V. N. (2011). Mesenchymal stromal cells in bronchoalveolar lavage as predictors of bronchiolitis obliterans syndrome. *American Journal of Respiratory and Critical Care Medicine*, *183*(8), 1062–1070. doi:10.1164/rccm.201005-0742OC

Banday, M. M., Kumar, A., Vestal, G., Sethi, J., Patel, K. N., O'Neill, E. B., & Sharma, N. S. (2021). N-myc-interactor mediates microbiome induced epithelial to mesenchymal transition and is associated with chronic lung allograft dysfunction. *The Journal of Heart and Lung Transplantation: The Official Publication of the International Society for Heart Transplantation*, *40*(6), 447–457. doi:10.1016/j.healun.2021.02.014

Bazemore, K., Rohly, M., Permpalung, N., Yu, K., Timofte, I., Brown, A. W., & Shah, P. D. (2021). Donor derived cell free DNA% is elevated with pathogens that are risk factors for acute and chronic lung allograft injury. *The Journal of Heart and Lung Transplantation: The Official Publication of the International Society for Heart Transplantation*, *40*(11), 1454–1462. doi:10.1016/j.healun.2021.05.012

Belperio, J., Palmer, S. M., & Weigt, S. S. (2017). Host-pathogen interactions and chronic lung allograft dysfunction. *Annals of the American Thoracic Society*, *14*(Suppl. 3), S242–S246. doi:10.1513/AnnalsATS.201606-464MG

Bernasconi, E., Pattaroni, C., Koutsokera, A., Pison, C., Kessler, R., Benden, C., & SysCLAD Consortium. (2016). Airway microbiota determines innate cell inflammatory or tissue remodeling profiles in lung transplantation. *American Journal of Respiratory and Critical Care Medicine*, *194*(10), 1252–1263. doi:10.1164/rccm.201512-2424OC

Berra, G., Farkona, S., Mohammed-Ali, Z., Kotlyar, M., Levy, L., Clotet-Freixas, S., & Martinu, T. (2021). Association between the renin-angiotensin system and chronic lung allograft dysfunction. *The European Respiratory Journal*, *58*(4), 2002975. doi:10.1183/13993003.02975-2020

Campos, S., Caramori, M., Teixeira, R., Afonso, J. J., Carraro, R., Strabelli, T., & Jatene, F. (2008a). Bacterial and fungal pneumonias after lung transplantation. *Transplantation Proceedings*, *40*(3), 822–824. doi:10.1016/j.transproceed.2008.02.049

Chambers, D. C., Perch, M., Zuckermann, A., Cherikh, W. S., Harhay, M. O., Hayes, D. J., & International Society for Heart and Lung Transplantation. (2021). The international thoracic organ transplant registry of the international society for heart and lung transplantation: Thirty-eighth adult lung transplantation report – 2021; focus on recipient characteristics. *The Journal of Heart and Lung Transplantation: The Official Publication of the International Society for Heart Transplantation*, *40*(10), 1060–1072. doi:10.1016/j.healun.2021.07.021

Combs, M. P., Wheeler, D. S., Luth, J. E., Falkowski, N. R., Walker, N. M., Erb-Downward, J. R., & Dickson, R. P. (2021). Lung microbiota predict chronic rejection in healthy lung transplant recipients: A prospective cohort study. *The Lancet Respiratory Medicine*, *9*(6), 601–612. doi:10.1016/S2213-2600(20)30405-7

Combs, M. P., Xia, M., Wheeler, D. S., Belloli, E. A., Walker, N. M., Braeuer, R. R., & Lama, V. N. (2020). Fibroproliferation in chronic lung allograft dysfunction: Association of mesenchymal cells in bronchoalveolar lavage with phenotypes and survival. *The Journal of Heart and Lung Transplantation: The Official Publication of the International Society for Heart Transplantation*, *39*(8), 815–823. doi:10.1016/j.healun.2020.04.011

Das, S., Bernasconi, E., Koutsokera, A., Wurlod, D., Tripathi, V., Bonilla-Rosso, G., & Nicod, L. P. (2021). A prevalent and culturable microbiota links ecological balance to clinical stability of the human lung after transplantation. *Nature Communications, 12*(1), 2126–4. doi:10.1038/s41467-021-22344-4

Du Rand, I. A., Blaikley, J. A. J., Booton, R., Chaudhuri, N., Gupta, V., Khalid, S., & British Thoracic Society Bronchoscopy Guideline Group. (2013). British thoracic society guideline for diagnostic flexible bronchoscopy in adults: Accredited by NICE. *Thorax, 68*(Suppl. 1), i1–i44. doi:10.1136/thoraxjnl-2013-203618

Engelmann, I., Welte, T., Fuhner, T., Simon, A. R., Mattner, F., Hoy, L., & Gottlieb, J. (2009). Detection of Epstein-Barr virus DNA in peripheral blood is associated with the development of bronchiolitis obliterans syndrome after lung transplantation. *Journal of Clinical Virology: The Official Publication of the Pan American Society for Clinical Virology, 45*(1), 47–53. doi:10.1016/j.jcv.2009.02.005

Girgis, R. E., Reichenspurner, H., Robbins, R. C., Reitz, B. A., & Theodore, J. (1995). The utility of annual surveillance bronchoscopy in heart-lung transplant recipients. *Transplantation, 60*(12), 1458–1461. doi:10.1097/00007890-199560120-00015

Glanville, A. R., Verleden, G. M., Todd, J. L., Benden, C., Calabrese, F., Gottlieb, J., & Snell, G. (2019). Chronic lung allograft dysfunction: Definition and update of restrictive allograft syndrome – A consensus report from the pulmonary council of the ISHLT. *The Journal of Heart and Lung Transplantation: The Official Publication of the International Society for Heart Transplantation, 38*(5), 483–492. doi:10.1016/j.healun.2019.03.008

Gottlieb, J., Schulz, T. F., Welte, T., Fuehner, T., Dierich, M., Simon, A. R., & Engelmann, I. (2009). Community-acquired respiratory viral infections in lung transplant recipients: A single season cohort study. *Transplantation, 87*(10), 1530–1537. doi:10.1097/TP.0b013e3181a4857d

Greenland, J. R., Jewell, N. P., Gottschall, M., Trivedi, N. N., Kukreja, J., Hays, S. R., & Caughey, G. H. (2014). Bronchoalveolar lavage cell immunophenotyping facilitates diagnosis of lung allograft rejection. *American Journal of Transplantation: Official Journal of the American Society of Transplantation and the American Society of Transplant Surgeons, 14*(4), 831–840. doi:10.1111/ajt.12630

Guilinger, R. A., Paradis, I. L., Dauber, J. H., Yousem, S. A., Williams, P. A., Keenan, R. J., & Griffith, B. P. (1995). The importance of bronchoscopy with transbronchial biopsy and bronchoalveolar lavage in the management of lung transplant recipients. *American Journal of Respiratory and Critical Care Medicine, 152*(6 Pt 1), 2037–2043. doi:10.1164/ajrccm.152.6.8520773

Haslam, P. L., & Baughman, R. P. (1999). Report of ERS task force: Guidelines for measurement of acellular components and standardization of BAL. *The European Respiratory Journal, 14*(2), 245–248. doi:10.1034/j.1399-3003.1999.14b01.x

Hayes, D. J., Benden, C., Sweet, S. C., & Conrad, C. K. (2015). Current state of pediatric lung transplantation. *Lung, 193*(5), 629–637. doi:10.1007/s00408-015-9765-z

Hayes, D. J., Cherikh, W. S., Harhay, M. O., Perch, M., Hsich, E., Potena, L., & International Society for Heart and Lung Transplantation. (2022). The international thoracic organ transplant registry of the international society for heart and lung transplantation: Twenty-fifth pediatric lung transplantation report – 2022; focus on pulmonary vascular diseases. *The Journal of Heart and Lung Transplantation: The Official Publication of the International Society for Heart Transplantation, 41*(10), 1348–1356. doi:10.1016/j.healun.2022.07.020

Iablonskii, P., Carlens, J., Mueller, C., Aburahma, K., Niehaus, A., Boethig, D., & Schwerk, N. (2022). Indications and outcome after lung transplantation in children under 12 years of age: A 16-year single center experience. *The Journal of Heart and Lung Transplantation:*

The Official Publication of the International Society for Heart Transplantation, 41(2), 226–236. doi:10.1016/j.healun.2021.10.012

Iasella, C. J., Hoji, A., Popescu, I., Wei, J., Snyder, M. E., Zhang, Y., & McDyer, J. F. (2021). Type-1 immunity and endogenous immune regulators predominate in the airway transcriptome during chronic lung allograft dysfunction. American Journal of Transplantation: Official Journal of the American Society of Transplantation and the American Society of Transplant Surgeons, 21(6), 2145–2160. doi:10.1111/ajt.16360

Inoue, M., Minami, M., Wada, N., Nakagiri, T., Funaki, S., Kawamura, T., & Okumura, M. (2014). Results of surveillance bronchoscopy after cadaveric lung transplantation: A japanese single-institution study. Transplantation Proceedings, 46(3), 944–947. doi:10.1016/j.transproceed.2013.10.055

Khan, M. S., Zhang, W., Taylor, R. A., Dean McKenzie, E., Mallory, G. B., Schecter, M. G., … Adachi, I. (2015). Survival in pediatric lung transplantation: The effect of center volume and expertise. The Journal of Heart and Lung Transplantation: The Official Publication of the International Society for Heart Transplantation, 34(8), 1073–1081. doi:10.1016/j.healun.2015.03.008

Levy, L., Tigert, A., Huszti, E., Saito, T., Mitsakakis, N., Moshkelgosha, S., & Martinu, T. (2019). Epithelial cell death markers in bronchoalveolar lavage correlate with chronic lung allograft dysfunction subtypes and survival in lung transplant recipients-a single-center retrospective cohort study. Transplant International: Official Journal of the European Society for Organ Transplantation, 32(9), 965–973. doi:10.1111/tri.13444

Martinu, T., Koutsokera, A., Benden, C., Cantu, E., Chambers, D., Cypel, M., & Bronchoalveolar Lavage Standardization Workgroup. (2020). International Society for Heart and Lung Transplantation consensus statement for the standardization of bronchoalveolar lavage in lung transplantation. The Journal of Heart and Lung Transplantation: The Official Publication of the International Society for Heart Transplantation, 39(11), 1171–1190. doi:10.1016/j.healun.2020.07.006

Meyer, K. C., Raghu, G., Baughman, R. P., Brown, K. K., Costabel, U., du Bois, R. M., & American Thoracic Society Committee on BAL in Interstitial Lung Disease. (2012). An official American Thoracic Society clinical practice guideline: The clinical utility of bronchoalveolar lavage cellular analysis in interstitial lung disease. American Journal of Respiratory and Critical Care Medicine, 185(9), 1004–1014. doi:10.1164/rccm.201202-0320ST

Neurohr, C., Huppmann, P., Samweber, B., Leuschner, S., Zimmermann, G., Leuchte, H., & Munich Lung Transplant Group. (2009). Prognostic value of bronchoalveolar lavage neutrophilia in stable lung transplant recipients. The Journal of Heart and Lung Transplantation: The Official Publication of the International Society for Heart Transplantation, 28(5), 468–474. doi:10.1016/j.healun.2009.01.014

Perch, M., Hayes, D. J., Cherikh, W. S., Zuckermann, A., Harhay, M. O., Hsich, E., & International Society for Heart and Lung Transplantation. (2022). The international thoracic organ transplant registry of the International Society for Heart and Lung Transplantation: Thirty-ninth adult lung transplantation report-2022; focus on lung transplant recipients with chronic obstructive pulmonary disease. The Journal of Heart and Lung Transplantation: The Official Publication of the International Society for Heart Transplantation, 41(10), 1335–1347. doi:10.1016/j.healun.2022.08.007

Reynaud-Gaubert, M., Thomas, P., Badier, M., Cau, P., Giudicelli, R., & Fuentes, P. (2000). Early detection of airway involvement in obliterative bronchiolitis after lung transplantation: Functional and bronchoalveolar lavage cell findings. American Journal of Respiratory and Critical Care Medicine, 161(6), 1924–1929. doi:10.1164/ajrccm.161.6.9905060

Saito, T., Liu, M., Binnie, M., Sato, M., Hwang, D., Azad, S., & Keshavjee, S. (2014). Distinct expression patterns of alveolar "alarmins" in subtypes of chronic lung allograft dysfunction. *American Journal of Transplantation: Official Journal of the American Society of Transplantation and the American Society of Transplant Surgeons, 14*(6), 1425–1432. doi:10.1111/ajt.12718

Schneck, E., Askevold, I., Rath, R., Hecker, A., Reichert, M., Guth, S., & Hecker, M. (2022). Chronic lung allograft dysfunction is associated with increased levels of cell-free mitochondrial DNA in bronchoalveolar lavage fluid of lung transplant recipients. *Journal of Clinical Medicine, 11*(14), 4142. doi: 10.3390/jcm11144142

Shino, M. Y., Weigt, S. S., Li, N., Derhovanessian, A., Sayah, D. M., Saggar, R., & Belperio, J. A. (2018). The prognostic importance of bronchoalveolar lavage fluid CXCL9 during minimal acute rejection on the risk of chronic lung allograft dysfunction. *American Journal of Transplantation: Official Journal of the American Society of Transplantation and the American Society of Transplant Surgeons, 18*(1), 136–144. doi:10.1111/ajt.14397

Shino, M. Y., Weigt, S. S., Li, N., Palchevskiy, V., Derhovanessian, A., Saggar, R., & Belperio, J. A. (2013). CXCR3 ligands are associated with the continuum of diffuse alveolar damage to chronic lung allograft dysfunction. *American Journal of Respiratory and Critical Care Medicine, 188*(9), 1117–1125. doi:10.1164/rccm.201305-0861OC

Shino, M. Y., Weigt, S. S., Li, N., Palchevskiy, V., Derhovanessian, A., Saggar, R., & Belperio, J. A. (2017). The prognostic importance of CXCR3 chemokine during organizing pneumonia on the risk of chronic lung allograft dysfunction after lung transplantation. *PLOS ONE, 12*(7), e0180281. doi:10.1371/journal.pone.0180281

Slebos, D., Postma, D. S., Koeter, G. H., Van Der Bij, W., Boezen, M., & Kauffman, H. F. (2004). Bronchoalveolar lavage fluid characteristics in acute and chronic lung transplant rejection. *The Journal of Heart and Lung Transplantation: The Official Publication of the International Society for Heart Transplantation, 23*(5), 532–540. doi:10.1016/j.healun.2003.07.004

Tikkanen, J., Lemstrom, K., Halme, M., Pakkala, S., Taskinen, E., & Koskinen, P. (2001). Cytological monitoring of peripheral blood, bronchoalveolar lavage fluid, and transbronchial biopsy specimens during acute rejection and cytomegalovirus infection in lung and heart–lung allograft recipients. *Clinical Transplantation, 15*(2), 77–88. doi:10.1034/j.1399-0012.2001.150201.x

Urso, A., Leiva-Juarez, M. M., Briganti, D. F., Aramini, B., Benvenuto, L., Costa, J., & D'Ovidio, F. (2021). Aspiration of conjugated bile acids predicts adverse lung transplant outcomes and correlates with airway lipid and cytokine dysregulation. *The Journal of Heart and Lung Transplantation: The Official Publication of the International Society for Heart Transplantation, 40*(9), 998–1008. doi:10.1016/j.healun.2021.05.007

Valentine, V. G., Gupta, M. R., Weill, D., Lombard, G. A., LaPlace, S. G., Seoane, L., … Dhillon, G. S. (2009). Single-institution study evaluating the utility of surveillance bronchoscopy after lung transplantation. *The Journal of Heart and Lung Transplantation: The Official Publication of the International Society for Heart Transplantation, 28*(1), 14–20. doi:10.1016/j.healun.2008.10.010

Vanaudenaerde, B. M., Meyts, I., Vos, R., Geudens, N., De Wever, W., Verbeken, E. K., … Verleden, G. M. (2008). A dichotomy in bronchiolitis obliterans syndrome after lung transplantation revealed by azithromycin therapy. *The European Respiratory Journal, 32*(4), 832–843. doi:10.1183/09031936.00134307

Vandermeulen, E., Lammertyn, E., Verleden, S. E., Ruttens, D., Bellon, H., Ricciardi, M., … Vanaudenaerde, B. M. (2017). Immunological diversity in phenotypes of chronic lung allograft dysfunction: A comprehensive immunohistochemical analysis. *Transplant International: Official Journal of the European Society for Organ Transplantation, 30*(2), 134–143. doi:10.1111/tri.12882

Vandermeulen, E., Verleden, S. E., Bellon, H., Ruttens, D., Lammertyn, E., Claes, S., ... Vanaudenaerde, B. M. (2016). Humoral immunity in phenotypes of chronic lung allograft dysfunction: A broncho-alveolar lavage fluid analysis. *Transplant Immunology, 38*, 27–32. doi:10.1016/j.trim.2016.08.004

Vandermeulen, E., Verleden, S. E., Ruttens, D., Moelants, E., Mortier, A., Somers, J., ... Vanaudenaerde, B. M. (2015). BAL neutrophilia in azithromycin-treated lung transplant recipients: Clinical significance. *Transplant Immunology, 33*(1), 37–44. doi:10.1016/j.trim.2015.07.001

Verleden, G. M., Glanville, A. R., Lease, E. D., Fisher, A. J., Calabrese, F., Corris, P. A., ... Vos, R. (2019). Chronic lung allograft dysfunction: Definition, diagnostic criteria, and approaches to treatment-A consensus report from the pulmonary council of the ISHLT. *The Journal of Heart and Lung Transplantation: The Official Publication of the International Society for Heart Transplantation, 38*(5), 493–503. doi:10.1016/j.healun.2019.03.009

Verleden, S. E., Hendriks, J. M. H., Lauwers, P., Yogeswaran, S. K., Verplancke, V., & Kwakkel-Van-Erp, J. M. (2023a). Biomarkers for chronic lung allograft dysfunction: Ready for prime time? *Transplantation, 107*(2), 341–350. doi:10.1097/TP.0000000000004270

Verleden, S. E., Hendriks, J. M. H., Lauwers, P., Yogeswaran, S. K., Verplancke, V., & Kwakkel-Van-Erp, J. M. (2023b). Biomarkers for chronic lung allograft dysfunction: Ready for prime time? *Transplantation, 107*(2), 341–350. doi:10.1097/TP.0000000000004270

Verleden, S. E., Ruttens, D., Vandermeulen, E., Bellon, H., Dubbeldam, A., De Wever, W., & Vos, R. (2016). Predictors of survival in restrictive chronic lung allograft dysfunction after lung transplantation. *The Journal of Heart and Lung Transplantation: The Official Publication of the International Society for Heart Transplantation, 35*(9), 1078–1084. doi:10.1016/j.healun.2016.03.022

Verleden, S. E., Ruttens, D., Vandermeulen, E., van Raemdonck, D. E., Vanaudenaerde, B. M., Verleden, G. M., & Vos, R. (2014). Elevated bronchoalveolar lavage eosinophilia correlates with poor outcome after lung transplantation. *Transplantation, 97*(1), 83–89. doi:10.1097/TP.0b013e3182a6bae2

Verleden, S. E., Ruttens, D., Vos, R., Vandermeulen, E., Moelants, E., Mortier, A., & Vanaudenaerde, B. M. (2015). Differential cytokine, chemokine and growth factor expression in phenotypes of chronic lung allograft dysfunction. *Transplantation, 99*(1), 86–93. doi:10.1097/TP.0000000000000269

Vos, R., Vanaudenaerde, B. M., Verleden, S. E., Ruttens, D., Vaneylen, A., Van Raemdonck, D. E., & Verleden, G. M. (2012). Anti-inflammatory and immunomodulatory properties of azithromycin involved in treatment and prevention of chronic lung allograft rejection. *Transplantation, 94*(2), 101–109. doi:10.1097/TP.0b013e31824db9da

Walts, A. E., Marchevsky, A. M., & Morgan, M. (1991). Pulmonary cytology in lung transplant recipients: Recent trends in laboratory utilization. *Diagnostic Cytopathology, 7*(4), 353–358. doi:10.1002/dc.2840070406

Wanner, T. J., Gerhardt, S. G., Diette, G. B., Rosenthal, D. L., & Orens, J. B. (2005). The utility of cytopathology testing in lung transplant recipients. *The Journal of Heart and Lung Transplantation: The Official Publication of the International Society for Heart Transplantation, 24*(7), 870–874. doi:10.1016/j.healun.2004.04.019

Watzenboeck, M. L., Gorki, A., Quattrone, F., Gawish, R., Schwarz, S., Lambers, C., & Knapp, S. (2022). Multi-omics profiling predicts allograft function after lung transplantation. *The European Respiratory Journal, 59*(2), 2003292. doi:10.1183/13993003.03292-2020

Weigt, S. S., Wang, X., Palchevskiy, V., Patel, N., Derhovanessian, A., Shino, M. Y., & Belperio, J. A. (2017). Gene expression profiling of bronchoalveolar lavage cells preceding a clinical diagnosis of chronic lung allograft dysfunction. *Annals of the American Thoracic Society, 14*(Suppl. 3), S252. doi:10.1513/AnnalsATS.201608-618MG

Wheeler, D. S., Misumi, K., Walker, N. M., Vittal, R., Combs, M. P., Aoki, Y., & Lama, V. N.

(2021). Interleukin 6 trans-signaling is a critical driver of lung allograft fibrosis. *American Journal of Transplantation: Official Journal of the American Society of Transplantation and the American Society of Transplant Surgeons, 21*(7), 2360–2371. doi:10.1111/ajt.16417

Yang, J. Y. C., Verleden, S. E., Zarinsefat, A., Vanaudenaerde, B. M., Vos, R., Verleden, G. M., & Sarwal, M. M. (2019). Cell-free DNA and CXCL10 derived from bronchoalveolar lavage predict lung transplant survival. *Journal of Clinical Medicine, 8*(2), 241. doi:10.3390/jcm8020241

12

Pediatric BAL

RICHARD WONG, DANIELLE MUNCE, DEHUA WANG, KELAN TANTISIRA, AND APARNA RAO

INSTRUMENTS

Bronchoalveolar lavage (BAL) is a procedure used to sample alveolar compartments for different cell types, biochemical components, and infectious pathogens. For pediatric patients, BAL is typically performed with a flexible fiberoptic bronchoscope which is introduced either through the nose or mouth. Available pediatric flexible bronchoscopes range from 2.2 to 6.3 mm in outer diameter (OD) with inner diameters that range from 1.2 to 3.2 mm. Selection of the appropriate size bronchoscope depends on the size of the patient's airway and the indication for bronchoscopy. In neonates, ultrathin bronchoscopes are available (2.2 mm OD), however these instruments are unable to accommodate suction channels, and therefore unable to perform lavage. Larger bronchoscopes (4.4–4.9 mm OD) are better suited for BAL given their larger suction channels.[1] Typically, these larger bronchoscopes can be used for school-aged children and adolescents. However, BAL can be performed in younger children with bronchoscopes as small as 2.7–2.8 mm OD, typically the smallest bronchoscopes with suction channels. To estimate the size of the patient's airway, the following calculation has been proposed: airway caliber (mm) = 4 + (age in years)/4. When choosing a bronchoscope in intubated patients, the size of the bronchoscope should be determined by the size of the endotracheal tube (ETT) since the bronchoscope will partially occlude the lumen of the ETT, which can affect ventilation or cause increased positive end expiratory pressure. Generally, the bronchoscope outer diameter should be at least less than 1 mm of the ETT inner diameter to allow for adequate ventilation during the procedure.[2]

TECHNIQUE

BAL is typically performed at a target region, based on imaging (combined with knowledge of bronchoscopic anatomy) or direct visualization, felt to best represent pathologic changes inside the affected lung. Additionally, samples can be obtained in multiple lobes to provide comprehensive microbiologic diversity.[19] If there is no specific targetable area, or in diffuse disease, the right middle lobe should be lavaged in children/adolescents and the right lower lobe in infants as they offer greater fluid recovery.[3–5] Once the

DOI: 10.1201/9781003146834-14

target area has been identified, the bronchoscope is gently wedged into the selected bronchus. BAL is then performed by instilling aliquots of normal saline through the working channel of the bronchoscope. There is limited evidence on the optimal amount of fluid needed for BAL in children of different ages and sizes. Given the lack of a universal protocol, the amount of saline used for lavage varies by center. Some bronchoscopists use 10–20 ml in 2–4 aliquots despite the patient's age and size, as in adults. Others adjust BAL volume to body weight using 3 ml/kg of normal saline divided into 3 aliquots with maximum volume of 20 ml/kg.[6] Fluid recovery can either be performed with a syringe by mechanical aspiration via a push-pull method or using wall suction to capture fluid in an inline trap. Both techniques yield equivalent return volumes of BAL samples.[7] The volume return requirement is often dictated by specific lab testing for a suspected diagnosis. A minimum volume of 5 ml is necessary for BAL cellular analysis.[8] BAL is considered successful if there is a return of at least 30–40% of the aliquot used in lavage,[5,9,10] along with evidence of surfactant in the sample. Return of 30% less than the instilled total fluid is suboptimal as the samples may provide inaccurate representations of the cell differential.[8]

BAL PROCESSING

Processing of bronchoalveolar lavage fluid (BALF) in pediatric patients does not differ from adult patients.[11] Once fluid has been obtained, differential cytology can be performed to establish the number of nucleated and red blood cells, as well as different types of white blood cells. Previous studies have revealed differential cytology of BALF in a healthy pediatric patient is similar to that of healthy adults, however younger children have a greater number of total cells when compared to adults. Similar to adults, macrophages are the predominant cell type recovered from BALF, typically 80–90% of all cell types, followed by lymphocytes. It has also been shown that the percentage of neutrophils is higher in sampled children less than 12 months of age compared to older children[12] (Figure 12.1). The major difference between pediatric and adult BALF is the CD4/CD8 ratio, which has been found to be lower in children with a mean of 0.7.[13,14] Elevation of this ratio may be suggestive of underlying pathology such as pulmonary sarcoidosis.

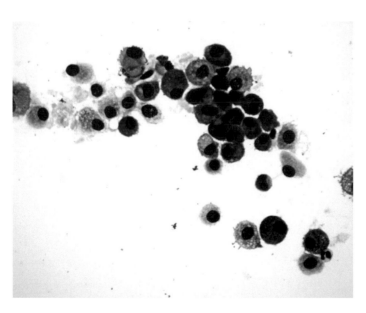

Figure 12.1 Normal BAL specimen. Predominant macrophages mixed with rare ciliated respiratory epithelial cells, neutrophils, and lymphocytes (Wright stain, 40×).

INFECTIOUS DISEASE

Flexible bronchoscopy (FB) and BAL are often utilized in infectious work-up involving both immunocompetent and immunocompromised patients. The goals of obtaining samples are to guide the diagnosis of causative pathogens causing pneumonia that will lead to treatment changes in promoting a more targeted antimicrobial therapy. This tool is particularly helpful in pediatrics or patients who are unable to expectorate to provide sputum culture. In children both in the United States and worldwide, pneumonia remains one of the leading causes of morbidity and mortality (Figures 12.2–12.3).

In immunocompetent hosts, community-acquired pneumonia is a heterogenous disease attributed to viral and bacterial infection. There are approximately 1.5 million pediatric cases annually.[15] Viral pathogens are the predominant cause of infection. The use of polymerase chain reaction (PCR) respiratory viral tests may account for increased incidence and detection. However, coinfection with superimposed bacterial pneumonia can occur as viral infection alters host defense systems leading to suboptimal clearance of airway pathogens and opportunity for bacterial growth.[16]

Obtaining samples for Gram stain and culture is indicated in persistent or recurrent episodes of pneumonia unresponsive to adequate empiric antimicrobial therapy. FB with BAL can not only assess disease severity, but also evaluate for anatomic airway anomalies that may make certain children more susceptible to developing recurrent, or persistent, pneumonia. BALF specimens obtained can be cultured, reviewed for cytology, and sent for immunofluorescence, nucleic acid amplification testing, sequencing, and PCR testing. Utilization of specialized media during culturing processes can allow for more expansive diagnostics. Cell count distribution of lymphocytes, neutrophils, and eosinophils may provide diagnostic estimation of viral, bacterial, or fungal and parasitic infections (Figure 12.4). Diagnostic yield for community-associated bacterial pneumonia ranges from 30–72%. Falsely negative absence or low counts of bacterial culture growth may suggest the pathogen is susceptible to current empiric antibiotic therapy or that infection is in the early stages to provide a significant response. Yield in ventilator-associated pneumonia has an increased sensitivity and specificity ranging from

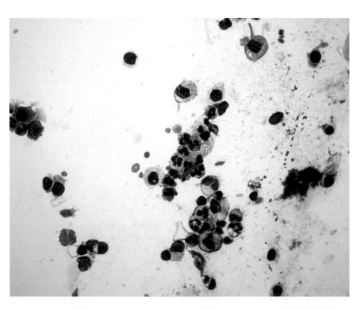

Figure 12.2 Acute inflammatory cells. BAL shows prominent neutrophils mixed with fewer macrophages and rare lymphocytes. Sample was obtained from a patient with bronchitis and pneumonia resulting in respiratory failure (Wright stain, 40×).

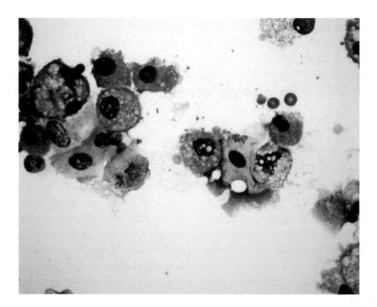

Figure 12.3 Intracellular and extracellular bacteria. BAL demonstrating macrophage, squamous epithelial cells, and intracellular and extracellular bacteria bacilli in a patient with normal respiratory flora confirmed on BAL culture (Wright stain, 60×).

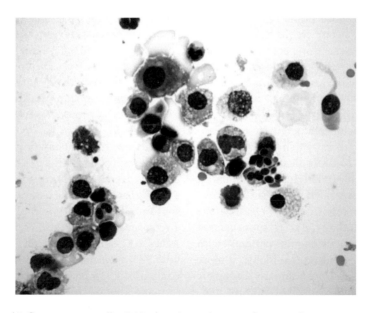

Figure 12.4 Mixed inflammatory cells. BAL showing mixture of macrophages, neutrophils, and clusters of oval-shaped fungal yeasts obtained from a patient with pneumonia and respiratory failure (Wright stain, 60×).

50–100% and 71–100%, respectively.[17] Utilization of culture data and labs from BAL has contributed to changes in antibiotic therapy in about 36–65% of patient cases in which BAL is performed.[18]

In immunocompromised patients, pulmonary infections can be resultant of underlying immunodeficiency or due to immunosuppressive therapies. BAL samples supplement diagnosis to help identify and differentiate new radiologic infiltrates between infection and medication or pathologic-related pulmonary disease. A retrospective review consisting of 198 pediatric cancer patients with suspected pneumonia underwent 264 total FB bronchoscopy cases. BAL was the most commonly documented indication among this population. In this study, BAL was able to yield positive cultures with a single pathogen identified in 60% of cases. This study also demonstrated greater volume of fluid instilled during the BAL procedure yielded a higher probability of positive culture results.[20] Pathogens involved in an immunocompromised host are much more diverse and multiple pathogens can occur simultaneously during an acute infection. Certain infections can lead to more prolonged and severe diseases requiring more supportive care and treatments due to impaired host immune response. Therefore, identification with samples obtained via BAL can be pivotal in implementing early targeted therapeutic regimens as these patients are more susceptible to infections. Treatment changes occur frequently based on BAL specimen results. A retrospective study evaluated 132 immunosuppressed children who had treatment changes with the escalation of therapy in approximately 90% of patients after implementing results obtained from BAL.[21]

BAL can be safely conducted in immunocompromised patients in which transbronchial lung biopsy may be contraindicated due to hemorrhagic risks from underlying coagulopathy. Peikert et al. demonstrated the utility of BAL results.[22] This study reported BAL results alone attributed to more than 50% of management changes in febrile neutropenia patients with radiologic pulmonary infiltrates. Biopsy, a more invasive procedure, did not increase diagnostic yield when supplemented by BAL culture findings.[22] BAL can be diagnostic of pneumonia when pathogens that should not be present in the lung are retrieved. This is critical in immunocompromised patients who need prompt antimicrobial interventions. In quantitative BAL cultures, a cut-off of $>10^4$ colony-forming units/ml can be utilized to distinguish bacterial pneumonia with high specificity.[23] BAL has been able to diagnose up to 64–68% of human stem cell transplant patients with pulmonary bacterial pneumonia allowing for tailored treatment to minimize post-implant infectious complications.[24]

Pulmonary fungal infections are more prevalent and can cause significant morbidity and mortality in immunocompromised hosts. Invasive pulmonary aspergillosis is one of the most common fungal infections in these patients and diagnostic BAL testing can allow for timely initiation of antifungal therapy. Timely diagnosis can lead to quicker treatments and higher success rates. US and European guidelines for diagnosis still lack a highly sensitive and specific test. Definitive diagnosis requires positive culture and identification of histopathology (Figure 12.5). Recent use of galactomannan assay, which tests for antigens from aspergillus cell walls, allows quicker testing results relative to fungal culture. This test has increased sensitivity and specificity for Aspergillus if detected in BALF in aiding diagnosis.[25] Additionally, PCR-based testing applied to BALF has high sensitivity. A combination of testing including galactomannan EIA with PCR or lateral flow assay testing can increase sensitivity to 94–100% without sacrificing testing specificity.[26]

Other opportunistic infections commonly affecting immunocompromised hosts include *Pneumocystis jirovecii*. Infections such as *Pneumocystis jirovecii* can pose life-threatening diseases in immunocompromised hosts leading to respiratory failure. Definitive diagnosis requires dye-based staining, fluorescent antibody staining, or PCR-based assays of BAL samples or sputum as pneumocystis cannot be cultured. In a retrospective study of 55 adults without HIV/AIDS, BAL samples were able to accurately diagnose 98% pneumocystis jirovecii pneumonia. In comparison, samples obtained from induced sputum and lung biopsy were diagnostic in 50% and 38%, respectively.[27]

Positive culture is often the primary diagnostic standard in diagnosing certain infections. However, positive yield on culture is dependent on the amount of living pathogens. Thus, diagnostic culture yields are often affected by pre-treatment of antimicrobials or early stages of infection that do not meet diagnostic cut-off values during the time of sampling, which can

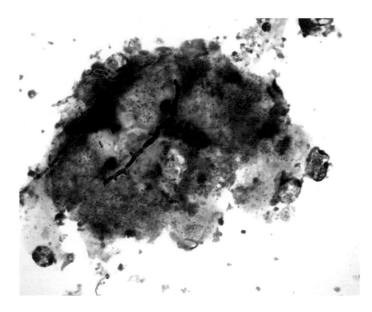

Figure 12.5 *Aspergillus fumigatus.* BAL showing fungal hyphae with septate and right-angle branching in the background of thick mucus material (Wright stain, 60×).

lead to false negative results. The introduction of multiplex PCR of BAL fluid has improved pathogen detection. Detection is more than doubled in PCR samples compared to traditional culture methods. These findings were both consistent in immunocompetent and immunosuppressed patients. However, one limitation of PCR testing is that it does not differentiate colonization vs active invasive infection.[28]

CHRONIC PULMONARY ASPIRATION

Chronic pulmonary aspiration often affects patients with underlying neurologic disease, premature infants with impaired swallowing mechanics, and patients with pharyngeal and airway anatomic abnormalities. As a result, oral secretions and gastric refluxate may penetrate the airway and lead to chronic lung disease with complications that may consist of chronic cough, recurrent pneumonia, wheezing, and failure to thrive. BAL can be useful in the assessment for diagnosis of chronic aspiration. FB can visually evaluate swallowing mechanics and airway penetration of the aspirate. Direct visualization for anatomic defects and inflammatory changes within the airway can also guide diagnosis.

BAL samples can be utilized to measure the lipid-laden macrophage index (LLMI), which is a sensitive marker of aspiration. Lipid-laden macrophages (LLMs) are biomarkers resultant of alveolar macrophages that phagocytize food particles as the respiratory system's innate defensive mechanism. The LLMI is graded from 0 to 4 based on the quantity of cytoplasmic lipid among 100 alveolar macrophages. While some studies suggest an LLMI greater than 100 indicates evidence of aspiration, there is no standardized consensus regarding a cut-off score[1] (Figure 12.6(a)–(b)). This testing modality is sensitive; however, it is unable to differentiate between exogenous and endogenous lipids, which may attribute to high false positive results. Beneficially, its ease of collection and measuring is a helpful diagnostic tool in patients with suspected aspiration.[29]

Tracheal pepsin is another biomarker for reflux aspiration. It is the active enzyme of the pepsinogen zymogen proenzyme. Pepsinogen is secreted by gastric chief cells that are activated by the gastric acidic environment; thus, its presence in BAL fluid collection has been shown to be sensitive and specific for pathologic reflux resulting in pulmonary aspiration. Measurement of gastric pepsin within the airway can provide guidance

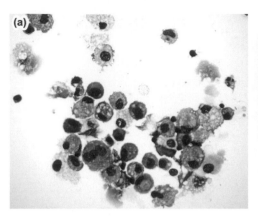
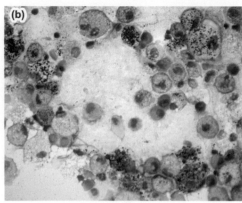

Figure 12.6 (a) Lipid-laden macrophages. BAL showing predominant macrophages, some of them appearing with foamy cytoplasm (Wright stain, 60×). (b) Lipid-laden macrophages. Oil-red-O staining showing macrophages with variable size and amount of lipid droplets and lipid-laden macrophage index 100 out of 400.

on the presence of aspiration; however, its use will need further investigation regarding diagnostic thresholds, collection timing, and location before implementation as a test for confirming diagnosis of pathologic reflux-associated aspiration.[30,31]

A-lactoalbumin and B-lactoglobulin are milk proteins that can be detected in immunocytochemical staining from BAL. Its use is currently limited to research in evaluating the presence of aspiration in murine models and infants.[32,33]

BAL IN PEDIATRIC PULMONARY HEMORRHAGE

The differential for pulmonary hemorrhage in pediatric patients is broad. Initial evaluation should be targeted at determining the source and etiology of bleeding, and include focused clinical history, physical exam, laboratory evaluation, and radiographic studies. FB is generally not necessary for the initial diagnosis or management of pulmonary hemorrhage, particularly in cases where the bleeding can be attributed to trauma, infection, known bronchiectasis, or in patients with tracheostomy. In the setting of acute, massive bleeding, rigid bronchoscopy can both facilitate ventilation and allow for better airway clearance with its much larger bore operating channels, compared to the 1.2–2.2 mm suction catheter on the pediatric flexible bronchoscope.[34] When bleeding is more occult, as in

diffuse alveolar hemorrhage syndromes, FB with lavage can be used to both confirm the presence of pulmonary hemorrhage as well as investigate underlying etiology if it remains unclear.

When FB is being done for the diagnostic assessment of pulmonary hemorrhage, the procedure should be ideally performed after acute bleeding has subsided, allowing for optimal evaluation of the tracheobronchial tree. When combined with BAL, FB can ideally sample distal acinar units to both confirm and assess for underlying etiology of pulmonary hemorrhage.[35]

When investigating for pulmonary alveolar hemorrhage, the flexible bronchoscope is wedged into the subsegmental bronchus of interest and aliquots of sterile saline are instilled, using suction to gather return. The optimal volume for lavage remains unclear, however most centers will use 10–20 ml-sized aliquots. Alveolar hemorrhage is classically confirmed by increasing hemorrhagic return with each aliquot.[6]

Regardless of the gross appearance of the BALF, lavage samples should be sent for patient-appropriate infectious work-up and serologic evaluations to evaluate for rheumatologic etiologies such as anti-neutrophilic cytoplasmic antibody (ANCA)-associated vasculitides. Cytology assessing for the presence of hemosiderin-laden macrophages is helpful for diagnosing the presence in diffuse alveolar hemorrhage, especially in cases without frank evidence of hemorrhagic

BALF or hemoptysis. Historically, various criteria have been used to diagnose pulmonary hemorrhage based on the presence of hemosiderin-laden macrophages (Figures 12.7(a)–(b), 12.8(a)–(b)). The Golde score was initially proposed in adult patients; it assigns a rank to hemosiderin content after examining 200 alveolar macrophages. A Golde score of 20–100 is considered mild-to-moderate pulmonary hemorrhage, whereas a score of >100 is considered severe.[36,37] A correlation between the percentage of hemosiderin-laden macrophages and Golde score was later observed and a >20% hemosiderin-laden content was regarded as diagnostic for pulmonary hemorrhage.[38] While these criteria have been applied to pediatric patients, both clinical criteria were studied and validated only in adults. One previous study looking at BAL specimens from pediatric patients proposed that a hemosiderin-laden macrophage (HLM) index of >36% carried the highest sensitivity and specificity, 1 and 0.96 respectively, for pulmonary hemorrhage in children.[39] The timing of collection also alters the sensitivity of BAL in diagnosing pulmonary hemorrhage. Simulated alveolar hemorrhage models have shown that HLMs do not appear until 3 days

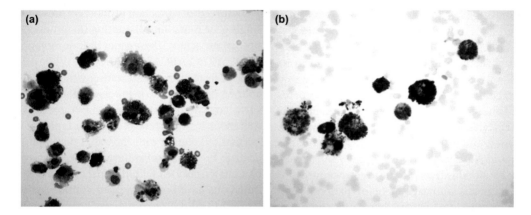

Figure 12.7 (a) Idiopathic pulmonary hemosiderosis. BAL demonstrating numerous macrophages with cytoplasmic dark brown granules consistent with hemosiderin-laden macrophages (Wright Stain, 60×). (b) Idiopathic pulmonary hemosiderosis. Iron stain (60×) confirming hemosiderin macrophages (iron stain, 60×).

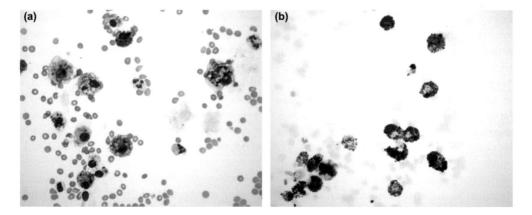

Figure 12.8 (a) Pulmonary capillaritis. BAL showing mainly hemosiderin-laden macrophages and RBCs (Wright stain, 60×). (b) Pulmonary capillaritis. Iron stain (60×) confirming hemosiderin-laden macrophages.

after hemorrhage, peak between 7–10 days, and continued to be present at 2 months.[40]

BAL IN CHILDHOOD INTERSTITIAL LUNG DISEASE

Childhood interstitial lung disease (chILD) refers to a heterogeneous group of disorders characterized by respiratory symptoms, diffuse lung disease, and impaired gas exchange. Unlike its name suggests, chILD affects not only the interstitial space but the airways and alveolar compartments as well. Compared to interstitial lung disease in adults, chILD is more diverse, comprising over 200 conditions, many of which are exclusive to the pediatric population. Despite its heterogeneity, chILD is a rare condition with most centers only seeing a few cases per year.[41] Given its overall rare prevalence, the first diagnostic step is to exclude other commonly recognized pediatric diffuse lung diseases, such as cystic fibrosis, primary ciliary dyskinesia, aspiration, immune deficiency, and infection. The chILD-EU collaboration and American Thoracic Society (ATS) have proposed standardized operating procedures for both diagnosis and treatment of patients with chILD. Alongside history, labs, and computed tomography imaging, FB with BAL is the most common invasive diagnostic technique used for diffuse lung disease given its relatively low contraindications and availability at most centers.[42] Both chILD-EU collaboration and ATS recommend the use of FB with BAL to rule out infection and airway anomalies as potential etiologies of diffuse lung disease.[43,44] Previous case series have shown that infection is the most common etiology for diffuse pulmonary infiltrates in children and diagnosis of a specific condition is rare.[45-47]

The sensitivity of BAL in diagnosing and monitoring disease activity is limited. However, the procedure can occasionally be diagnostic for specific conditions such as pulmonary alveolar proteinosis (PAP). PAP is a rare disorder of surfactant homeostasis characterized by accumulation of proteinaceous material in the alveoli. It can be caused by disorders of surfactant clearance, as well as deficiencies in surfactant production. In disorders of surfactant clearance, BAL is the key to diagnosis. BALF will typically reveal a classically "milky" fluid appearance on visual inspection.

Under light microscopy, fluid is notable for foamy macrophages and abundant globules of amorphous material that are Periodic acid-Schiff (PAS) stain positive. There are other causes of PAP including autoimmune disease with autoantibodies to granulocyte-macrophage colony stimulating factor blocking, which blocks activation of alveolar macrophages. PAS-positive cells have also been seen non-specifically in other forms of ILD, including sarcoidosis and idiopathic pulmonary fibrosis.[48,49] While BALF appearance and cytology may be indicative of PAP (Figure 12.9(a)–(b)). The majority of pediatric patients undergo lung biopsy to histologically confirm diagnosis of PAP.[50]

Disorders of surfactant production are caused by single gene mutations disrupting the production of normal surfactant. These genes include mutations in *SFTB*, *SFTPC*, *ABCA3*, and *NKX2.1*. While diagnosis relies heavily on genetic testing at this time, BALF analysis can be used to help support the diagnosis of surfactant dysfunction. The BALF of patients with mutations in surfactant production typically show normal cell counts with increased neutrophil percentage. Previous studies have revealed that western blot analysis of BALF fluid in patients with *SFTPC* mutations have both decreased mature Surfactant Protein C (SP-C) protein as well as accumulation of SP-C precursors. Elevation in SP-C precursors has been seen in patients with *SFTPB* and *ABCA3* mutations, as both mutations affect protein C processing and metabolism.[51] Mature Surfactant Protein-B (SP-B) levels are undetectable in the BALF of patients with *SFTB* mutations and normal with *SFTPC* mutations, however pro-SP-B profiles are typically abnormal in both. At this time, these assays are not widely available at all centers.

Alterations to normal BALF differential, while often non-specific, can support certain diagnoses. Normal cell differential in BALF reveals a predominance of macrophages followed by lymphocytes. In hypersensitivity pneumonitis (HP), acute antigen exposure is associated with an increase in neutrophils in BALF, followed by a lymphocytic alveolitis with lymphocytes comprising greater than 60% of cell differential.[52,53] In adult patients, BALF lymphocytosis with a decrease in the CD4:CD8 ratio has been classically associated with HP. While previous cases have similarly shown low CD4:CD8 ratios in the BALF of pediatric patients with HP, these were

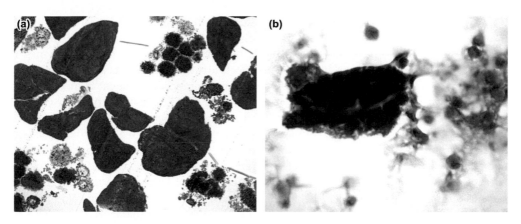

Figure 12.9 (a) Pulmonary alveolar proteinosis. BAL showing abundant dense eosinophilic protein-aceous material (Wright stain, 40×). Sample obtained from a patient with chronic interstitial lung disease/pulmonary alveolar proteinosis and immune dysregulation. (b) Pulmonary alveolar pro-teinosis. PAS-positive proteinaceous material (PAS stain, 60×). Sample obtained from a patient with chronic interstitial lung disease/pulmonary alveolar proteinosis and immune dysregulation.

based on adult reference values.[54,55] In studies of children without lung disease, it was found that CD4:CD8 ratios are normally lower than those of healthy adults.[14] A more recent study specifi-cally looking at BAL profiles of children of 6–15 years with HP revealed no significant difference between CD4:CD8 ratios between normal con-trols and patients with HP.[56]

In pulmonary sarcoidosis, BALF lymphocy-tosis with an increased CD4:CD8 ratio of more than 3.5:1 is associated with a diagnosis of pulmo-nary sarcoidosis, seen in 50–60% of patients.[57,58] Conversely, lymphocytosis with predominant CD8 cells in BALF is associated with connec-tive tissue disease and pulmonary histiocytosis. Eosinophilia (>25%) in BALF may also be indica-tive of underlying eosinophilic lung disease such as eosinophilic pneumonia, eosinophilic vasculi-tis, or processes like drug-induced pneumonitis[59] (Figure 12.10).

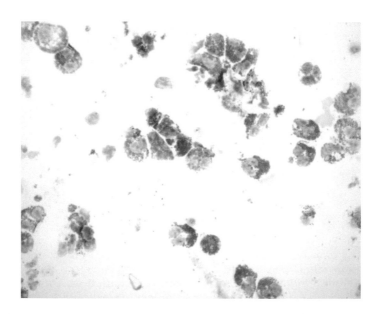

Figure 12.10 Pulmonary eosinophilia. BAL showing numerous eosinophils (Wright stain, 60×).

CARDIAC/PEDIATRIC INTENSIVE CARE

Congenital heart disease has a worldwide incidence of 12 per 1,000 live births.[60] Due to abnormal cardiac anatomy or surgical corrections to allow for proper cardiac physiology, the respiratory system may be impacted. The indications for FB with BAL in children with congenital heart disease include assisting with diagnosis of infection, therapeutic removal of proteinaceous airway debris to optimize and improve gas exchange and assist with diagnosis of non-infectious airway and lung disease.[61] Samples obtained from BAL can provide objective data on cellular activity including biologic and immunologic markers of certain disease to help guide therapy.

The incidence of hospital-acquired infections in children after cardiac surgery varies from 9.6 to 21.5%, which may require intensive care. Common pathogens are Gram-negative bacilli such as *Pseudomonas aeruginosa* and *Acinetobacter baumanii* followed by fungi, particularly *Candida albicans*, especially with prolonged hospital stays.[62,63]

Atelectasis is a common problem that is encountered in intensive care units. This is often related to airway pathologies that may include airway malacia, airway compression, or poor ciliary function.[64,65] There are also post-operative risk factors that place a patient at increased risk of atelectasis.

Additionally, patients who are critically ill are placed supine and immobilized and are given narcotics that suppress coughing, which negatively affects airway clearance. As a result of suboptimal airway clearance, the patient is more susceptible to mucus plugging that contributes to atelectasis, which can develop into infection. Neonates are particularly sensitive to alveolar collapse because of their small airway size and reduced number of interalveolar pores of Kohn and bronchiole-alveolar channels of Lambert.[66] While diagnostic BAL primarily assists with microbiologic cultures to guide antimicrobial therapies, it can have therapeutic interventions, which include re-expansion of persisting atelectasis, airway hemostasis, and removal of airway mucus plugs or casts.[61]

BAL is helpful in management of plastic bronchitis and cast bronchitis. Palliative univentricular Fontan physiology is associated with passive non-pulsatile drainage to the pulmonary arteries. Plastic bronchitis (PB) is a life-threatening airway obstruction due to cast formation in tracheobronchial tree. PB is rare, but it is a frequent occurrence in patients with single ventricle cardiac physiology who have undergone Fontan procedures. Casts may be composed of fibrinous material with eosinophilic infiltrates in patients with inflammatory pulmonary disease or may be acellular with mucin and no acute inflammatory cells in patients with cardiovascular disease [67] (Figure 12.11(a)–(b)). While small casts

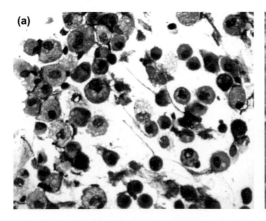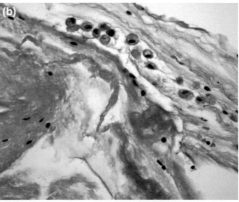

Figure 12.11 (a) Plastic bronchitis. A patient with congenital heart disease corrected with Fontan procedure with development of plastic bronchitis. BAL showing numerous macrophages mixed with proteinaceous debris (Wright stain, 40×). (b) Plastic bronchitis. A patient with congenital heart disease corrected with Fontan procedure with development of plastic bronchitis. Removed right bronchial cast demonstrates abundant proteinaceous material mixed with mucin, macrophages, and chronic inflammatory cells (H&E stain, 40×).

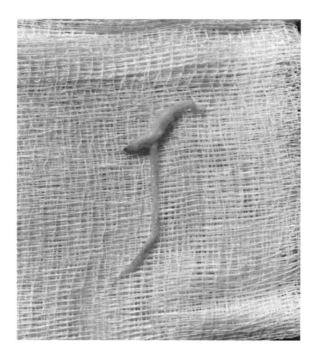

Figure 12.12 Surgically removed plastic bronchitis cast.

can be expectorated, large cast formations may require FB and lavage to assist with administration of mucolytics via irrigation and suctioning to extract cast occlusions. If unsuccessful, rigid bronchoscopy may be necessary for cast removal in these patients (Figure 12.12). Cast bronchitis is not only limited to cardiac abnormalities as it has also been reported in cases of sickle cell disease, primary lymphatic abnormalities, severe asthma, viral infections such as H1N1 influenza and COVID-19, and chronic lung diseases. BAL has diagnostic utility in guiding treatments by providing information regarding cytology that helps to classify and identify the etiology of patient disease that may attribute to cast formation. BAL also has therapeutic utility in alveolar lavage of medications that may be helpful in treating and removing certain types of cast bronchitis.[67,68]

PEDIATRIC LUNG TRANSPLANTATION

With approximately 100 lung transplants reported per year to the Registry of the International Society of Heart and Lung Transplantation, pediatric lung transplant is an uncommon procedure that provides a treatment option to eligible patients with end-stage lung disease.[69] The International Society for Heart and Lung Transplant has provided insight into the standardization of pediatric BAL procedure and processing as protocols vary within each lung transplant center. Some of these surveyed practices for BAL include 1 ml/kg instillation per aliquot with a maximum of 50 ml of sterile saline. There is a preference for immediate manual suctioning of BALF with no dwell time. BAL should also be performed prior to transbronchial biopsy (TBBx).[70]

Post lung transplant long-term survival remains inferior in comparison to other solid organ transplants. Common post-transplant complications that can cause death are graft failure and infection. Surveillance for graft rejection and infection is conducted with FB, BAL, and TBBx at set intervals in the first year after transplantation. Allograft rejections present similarly to pulmonary infection; therefore, FB with BAL is clinically indicated outside of planned surveillance procedures to guide diagnosis and treatment.[69,71]

Visualization with FB can assess bronchial anastomoses, areas of airway malacia, and mucosal changes that are unable to be conducted with radiographic imaging. TBBx can also be conducted to evaluate the healing process or presence of graft rejection.[72]

Many of these patients are medically immunosuppressed to mitigate graft rejection and are therefore susceptible to infection. Additional infection risk factors related to transplantation include infection in the donor organ prior to transplantation, impairment of pulmonary lymphatic flow, ineffective cough, recipient airway colonization, and suboptimal mucociliary movement and clearance at the site of anastomosis. BAL is primarily utilized to evaluate and diagnose for infections, which include bacteria, fungi, and mycobacteria. Immunofluorescence testing aids in the detection of cytomegalovirus, adenovirus, parainfluenza virus, respiratory syncytial virus, and *Pneumocystis jirovecii*. Utilization of PCR testing has increased sensitivity of pathogen detection.[69,70]

BAL analysis needs to include total cell and differential counts as it provides information regarding the status of transplantation allograft. Differential cytology evolves from the early to late transplantation period. Initially, total cell counts are elevated with a neutrophilic alveolitis that reflects cellular response to lung graft injury. There is a shift to lower CD4 cells in BALF in the later transplantation period. Persistent neutrophilia can be utilized as a predictive prognostic marker for bronchiolitis obliterans syndrome, which can be a chronic complication of lung transplantation.[73]

CONCLUSION

In pediatrics, BAL can be successfully performed in all but the very youngest/smallest of children. BAL is used in a wide variety of clinical settings both for diagnosis and therapy. In addition to the clinical applications for BAL, the technique is increasingly being applied in research settings, where in addition to cellular and microbiologic analyses, isolation of DNA, RNA, proteins, surfactants, and other biomarkers can be readily applied to lung disease research in children.[74] Moreover, state-of-the-art molecular approaches, such as single cell RNA-sequencing, have begun

to identify subsets of cells that may uniquely influence outcomes in community-acquired pneumonia in children. Thus, BAL will continue to play a key role in pediatric clinical care, research diagnostics, and therapeutic developments now and for the foreseeable future.[75]

REFERENCES

1. Faro A, Wood RE, Schechter MS, et al. Official American Thoracic Society technical standards: Flexible airway endoscopy in children. *Am J Respir Crit Care Med* 2015;191(9):1066–1080. doi:10.1164/rccm.201503-0474ST

2. Wang KP, Mehta A. *Flexible Bronchoscopy.* 4th ed. Wiley-Blackwell; 2020.

3. Pohunek P, Pokorná H, Stríz I. Comparison of cell profiles in separately evaluated fractions of bronchoalveolar lavage (BAL) fluid in children. *Thorax* 1996;51(6):615–618. doi:10.1136/thx.51.6.615

4. Baughman RP. Technical aspects of bronchoalveolar lavage: Recommendations for a standard procedure. *Semin Respir Crit Care Med* 2007;28(5):475–485. doi:10.1055/s-2007-991520

5. de Blic J, Midulla F, Barbato A, et al. Bronchoalveolar lavage in children. ERS Task Force on Bronchoalveolar lavage in children. European Respiratory Society. *Eur Respir J* 2000;15(1):217–231. doi:10.1183/09031936.00.15121700

6. Ratjen F, Bruch J. Adjustment of bronchoalveolar lavage volume to body weight in children. *Pediatr Pulmonol* 1996;21(3):184–188. doi:10.1002/(SICI)1099-0496(199603)21:3<184::AID-PPUL6>3.0.CO;2-Q

7. Radhakrishna N, Farmer M, Steinfort DP, King P. *A Comparison of Techniques for Optimal Performance of Bronchoalveolar Lavage*; 2015. www.bronchology.com.

8. Meyer KC, Raghu G, Baughman RP, et al. An official American Thoracic Society clinical practice guideline: The clinical utility of bronchoalveolar lavage cellular analysis in interstitial lung disease. *Am J Respir Crit Care Med* 2012;185(9):1004–1014. doi:10.1164/rccm.201202-0320ST

9. Nicolai T. Pediatric bronchoscopy. *Pediatr Pulmonol* 2001;31(2):150–164. doi:10.100 2/1099-0496(200102)31:2<150::aid-pp ul1024>3.0.co;2-6

10. Baughman RP, Spencer RE, Kleykamp BO, Rashkin MC, Douthit MM. Ventilator associated pneumonia: Quality of nonbronchoscopic bronchoalveolar lavage sample affects diagnostic yield. *Eur Respir J* 2000;16(6):1152–1157. doi:10.1034/j.1399-3003.2000.16f23.x

11. Technical recommendations and guidelines for bronchoalveolar lavage (BAL). Report of the European Society of Pneumology task group. *Eur Respir J* 1989;2(6):561–585.

12. Midulla F, Villani A, Merolla R, Bjermer L, Sandstrom T, Ronchetti R. Bronchoalveolar lavage studies in children without parenchymal lung disease: Cellular constituents and protein levels. *Pediatr Pulmonol* 1995;20(2):112–118. doi:10.1002/ppul.1950200211

13. Riedler J, Grigg J, Stone C, Tauro G, Robertson CF. Bronchoalveolar lavage cellularity in healthy children. *Am J Respir Crit Care Med* 1995;152(1):163–168. doi:10.1164/ajrccm.152.1.7599817

14. Ratjen F, Bredendiek M, Zheng L, Brendel M, Costabel U. Lymphocyte subsets in bronchoalveolar lavage fluid of children without bronchopulmonary disease. *Am J Respir Crit Care Med* 1995;152(1):174–178. doi:10.1164/ajrccm.152.1.7599820

15. Kronman MP, Hersh AL, Feng R, Huang YS, Lee GE, Shah SS. Ambulatory visit rates and antibiotic prescribing for children with pneumonia, 1994–2007. *Pediatrics* 2011;127(3):411–418. doi:10.1542/peds.2010-2008

16. Bakaletz LO. Viral–bacterial co-infections in the respiratory tract. *Curr Opin Microbiol* 2017;35:30–35. doi:10.1016/j.mib.2016.11.003

17. Sanchez Nieto JM, Carillo Alcaraz A. *The Role of Bronchoalveolar Lavage in the Diagnosis of Bacterial Pneumonia*, Vol. 14; 1995.

18. Shorr AF, Sherner JH, Jackson WL, Kollef MH. Invasive approaches to the diagnosis of ventilator-associated pneumonia: A meta-analysis. *Crit Care Med* 2005;33(1):46–53. doi:10.1097/01.ccm.0000149852.32599.31

19. Gilchrist FJ, Salamat S, Clayton S, Peach J, Alexander J, Lenney W. Bronchoalveolar lavage in children with cystic fibrosis: How many lobes should be sampled? *Arch Dis Child* 2011;96(3):215–217. doi:10.1136/adc.2009.177618

20. Ahmad AH, Brown BD, Andersen CR, et al. Retrospective review of flexible bronchoscopy in pediatric cancer patients. *Front Oncol* 2021;11:770523. doi:10.3389/fonc.2021.770523

21. Eroglu-Ertugrul NG, Yalcin E, Oguz B, et al. The value of flexible bronchoscopy in pulmonary infections of immunosuppressed children. *Clin Respir J* 2020;14(2):78–84. doi:10.1111/crj.13103

22. Peikert T, Rana S, Edell ES. Safety, diagnostic yield, and therapeutic implications of flexible bronchoscopy in patients with febrile neutropenia and pulmonary infiltrates. *Mayo Clin Proc* 2005;80(11):1414–1420. doi:10.4065/80.11.1414

23. Rasmussen TR, Korsgaard J, Møller JK, Sommer T, Kilian M. Quantitative culture of bronchoalveolar lavage fluid in community-acquired lower respiratory tract infections. *Respir Med* 2001;95(11):885–890. doi:10.1053/rmed.2001.1160

24. Kasow KA, King E, Rochester R, et al. Diagnostic yield of bronchoalveolar lavage is low in allogeneic hematopoietic stem cell recipients receiving immunosuppressive therapy or with acute graft-versus-host disease: The St. Jude experience, 1990–2002. *Biol Blood Marrow Transplant* 2007;13(7):831–837. doi:10.1016/j.bbmt.2007.03.008

25. Zou M, Tang L, Zhao S, et al. Systematic review and meta-analysis of detecting galactomannan in bronchoalveolar lavage fluid for diagnosing invasive aspergillosis. *PLOS ONE* 2012;7(8):e43347. doi:10.1371/journal.pone.0043347

26. Hoenigl M, Prattes J, Spiess B, et al. Performance of galactomannan, beta-d-glucan, Aspergillus lateral-flow device, conventional culture, and PCR tests with bronchoalveolar lavage fluid for diagnosis of invasive pulmonary aspergillosis. *J Clin Microbiol* 2014;52(6):2039–2045. doi:10.1128/JCM.00467-14

27. Pagano L, Fianchi L, Mele L, et al. *Pneumocystis carinii* pneumonia in patients with malignant haematological diseases: 10 years' experience of infection in GIMEMA centres. *Br J Haematol* 2002;117(2):379–386. doi:10.1046/j.1365-2141.2002.03419.x

28. Tschiedel E, Goralski A, Steinmann J, et al. Multiplex PCR of bronchoalveolar lavage fluid in children enhances the rate of pathogen detection. *BMC Pulm Med* 2019;19(1):132. doi:10.1186/s12890-019-0894-7

29. Corwin RW, Irwin RS. The lipid-laden alveolar macrophage as a marker of aspiration in parenchymal lung disease. *Am Rev Respir Dis* 1985;132(3):576–581. doi:10.1164/arrd.1985.132.3.576

30. Farrell S, McMaster C, Gibson D, Shields MD, McCallion WA. Pepsin in bronchoalveolar lavage fluid: A specific and sensitive method of diagnosing gastro-oesophageal reflux-related pulmonary aspiration. *J Pediatr Surg* 2006;41(2):289–293. doi:10.1016/j.jpedsurg.2005.11.002

31. Calvo-Henríquez C, Ruano-Ravina A, Vaamonde P, Martínez-Capoccioni G, Martín-Martín C. Is pepsin A reliable marker of laryngopharyngeal reflux? A systematic review. *Otolaryngol Head Neck Surg* 2017;157(3):385–391. doi:10.1177/0194599817709430

32. Elidemir O, Fan LL, Colasurdo GN. A novel diagnostic method for pulmonary aspiration in a murine model. Immunocytochemical staining of milk proteins in alveolar macrophages. *Am J Respir Crit Care Med* 2000;161(2 Pt 1):622–626. doi:10.1164/ajrccm.161.2.9906036

33. de Baets F, Aarts C, van Daele S, et al. Milk protein and Oil-Red-O staining of alveolar macrophages in chronic respiratory disease of infancy. *Pediatr Pulmonol* 2010;45(12):1213–1219. doi:10.1002/ppul.21310

34. Karmy-Jones R, Cuschieri J, Vallières E. Role of bronchoscopy in massive hemoptysis. *Chest Surg Clin N Am* 2001;11(4):873–906.

35. Batra PS, Holinger LD. Etiology and management of pediatric hemoptysis. *Arch Otolaryngol Head Neck Surg* 2001;127(4):377. doi:10.1001/archotol.127.4.377

36. Golde DW, Drew WL, Klein HZ, Finley TN, Cline MJ. Occult pulmonary haemorrhage in leukaemia. *Br Med J* 1975;2(5964):166–168. doi:10.1136/bmj.2.5964.166

37. Maldonado F, Parambil JG, Yi ES, Decker PA, Ryu JH. Haemosiderin-laden macrophages in the bronchoalveolar lavage fluid of patients with diffuse alveolar damage. *Eur Respir J* 2009;33(6):1361–1366. doi:10.1183/09031936.00119108

38. Lauque D, Cadranel J, Lazor R, et al. Microscopic polyangiitis with alveolar hemorrhage. A study of 29 cases and review of the literature. Groupe d'Etudes et de Recherche sur les Maladies "Orphelines" Pulmonaires (GERM"O"P). *Medicine* 2000;79(4):222–233. doi:10.1097/00005792-200007000-00003

39. Salih ZN, Akhter A, Akhter J. Specificity and sensitivity of hemosiderin-laden macrophages in routine bronchoalveolar lavage in children. *Arch Pathol Lab Med* 2006;130(11):1684–1686. doi:10.5858/2006-130-1684-SASOHM

40. Epstein CE, Elidemir O, Colasurdo GN, Fan LL. Time course of hemosiderin production by alveolar macrophages in a murine model. *Chest* 2001;120(6):2013–2020. doi:10.1378/chest.120.6.2013

41. Cunningham S, Jaffe A, Young LR. Children's interstitial and diffuse lung disease. *Lancet Child Adolesc Health* 2019;3(8):568–577. doi:10.1016/S2352-4642(19)30117-8

42. Barbato A, Panizzolo C, Cracco A, de Blic J, Dinwiddie R, Zach M. Interstitial lung disease in children: A multicentre survey on diagnostic approach. *Eur Respir J* 2000;16(3):509–513. doi:10.1034/j.1399-3003.2000.016003509.x

43. Bush A, Cunningham S, de Blic J, et al. European protocols for the diagnosis and initial treatment of interstitial lung disease in children. *Thorax* 2015;70(11):1078–1084. doi:10.1136/thoraxjnl-2015-207349

44. Kurland G, Deterding RR, Hagood JS, et al. An official American Thoracic Society clinical practice guideline: Classification, evaluation, and management of childhood interstitial lung disease in infancy. *Am J Respir Crit Care Med* 2013;188(3):376–394. doi:10.1164/rccm.201305-0923ST

45. Riedler J, Grigg J, Robertson CF. Role of bronchoalveolar lavage in children with lung disease. *Eur Respir J* 1995;8(10):1725–1730. doi:10.1183/09031936.95.08101725

46. Rock MJ. The diagnostic utility of bronchoalveolar lavage in immunocompetent children with unexplained infiltrates on chest radiograph. *Pediatrics* 1995;95(3):373–377.

47. Fan LL, Lung MC, Wagener JS. The diagnostic value of bronchoalveolar lavage in immunocompetent children with chronic diffuse pulmonary infiltrates. *Pediatr Pulmonol* 1997;23(1):8–13. doi:10.1002/(sici)1099-0496(199701)23:1<8::aid-ppul1>3.0.co;2-n

48. Chou CW, Lin FC, Tung SM, Liou RD, Chang SC. Diagnosis of pulmonary alveolar proteinosis: Usefulness of Papanicolaou-stained smears of bronchoalveolar lavage fluid. *Arch Intern Med* 2001;161(4):562. doi:10.1001/archinte.161.4.562

49. Hauber HP, Zabel P. PAS staining of bronchoalveolar lavage cells for differential diagnosis of interstitial lung disease. *Diagn Pathol* 2009;4:13. doi:10.1186/1746-1596-4-13

50. Griese M. Pulmonary alveolar proteinosis: A comprehensive clinical perspective. *Pediatrics* 2017;140(2):e20170610. doi:10.1542/peds.2017-0610

51. Hildebrandt J, Yalcin E, Bresser HG, et al. Characterization of CSF2RA mutation related juvenile pulmonary alveolar proteinosis. *Orphanet J Rare Dis* 2014;9:171. doi:10.1186/s13023-014-0171-z

52. Spagnolo P, Rossi G, Cavazza A, et al. Hypersensitivity pneumonitis: A comprehensive review. *J Investig Allergol Clin Immunol* 2015;25(4):237–250; quiz follow 250.

53. Selman M, Buendía-Roldán I. Immunopathology, diagnosis, and management of hypersensitivity pneumonitis. *Semin Respir Crit Care Med* 2012;33(5):543–554. doi:10.1055/s-0032-1325163

54. Grech V, Vella C, Lenicker H. Pigeon breeder's lung in childhood: Varied clinical picture at presentation. *Pediatr Pulmonol* 2000;30(2):145–148. doi:10.1002/1099-0496(200008)30:2<145::AID-PPUL10>3.0.CO;2-4

55. du Marchie Sarvaas GJ, Merkus PJ, de Jongste JC. A family with extrinsic allergic alveolitis caused by wild city pigeons: A case report. *Pediatrics* 2000;105(5):E62. doi:10.1542/peds.105.5.e62

56. Ratjen F, Costabel U, Griese M, Paul K. Bronchoalveolar lavage fluid findings in children with hypersensitivity pneumonitis. *Eur Respir J* 2003;21(1):144–148. doi:10.1183/09031936.03.00035703a

57. Végh J, Soós G, Csipő I, et al. Pulmonary arterial hypertension in mixed connective tissue disease: Successful treatment with iloprost. *Rheumatol Int* 2006;26(3):264–269. doi:10.1007/s00296-005-0616-8

58. Baculard A, Blanc N, Boulé M, et al. Pulmonary sarcoidosis in children: A follow-up study. *Eur Respir J* 2001;17(4):628–635. doi:10.1183/09031936.01.17406280

59. Cottin V, Cordier JF. Eosinophilic pneumonias. *Allergy* 2005;60(7):841–857. doi:10.1111/j.1398-9995.2005.00812.x

60. Hoffman JI. Incidence of congenital heart disease: I. Postnatal incidence. *Pediatr Cardiol* 1995;16(3):103–113. doi:10.1007/BF00801907

61. Cerda J, Chacón J, Reichhard C, et al. Flexible fiberoptic bronchoscopy in

children with heart diseases: A twelve years experience. *Pediatr Pulmonol* 2007;42(4):319–324. doi:10.1002/ppul.20577

62. Tan L, Sun X, Zhu X, Zhang Z, Li J, Shu Q. Epidemiology of nosocomial pneumonia in infants after cardiac surgery. *Chest* 2004;125(2):410–417. doi:10.1378/chest.125.2.410

63. Fischer JE, Allen P, Fanconi S. Delay of extubation in neonates and children after cardiac surgery: Impact of ventilator-associated pneumonia. *Intensive Care Med* 2000;26(7):942–949. doi:10.1007/s001340051285

64. Healy F, Hanna BD, Zinman R. Pulmonary complications of congenital heart disease. *Paediatr Respir Rev* 2012;13(1):10–15. doi:10.1016/j.prrv.2011.01.007

65. Adams PS, Corcoran TE, Lin JH, Weiner DJ, Sanchez-de-Toledo J, Lo CW. Mucociliary clearance scans show infants undergoing congenital cardiac surgery have poor airway clearance function. *Front Cardiovasc Med* 2021;8. doi:10.3389/fcvm.2021.652158

66. Terry PB, Traystman RJ. The clinical significance of collateral ventilation. *Ann Am Thorac Soc* 2016;13(12):2251–2257. doi:10.1513/AnnalsATS.201606-448FR

67. Seear M, Hui H, Magee F, Bohn D, Cutz E. Bronchial casts in children: A proposed classification based on nine cases and a review of the literature. *Am J Respir Crit Care Med* 1997;155(1):364–370. doi:10.1164/ajrccm.155.1.9001337

68. Liptzin DR, McGraw MD, Houin PR, Veress LA. Fibrin airway cast obstruction: Experience, classification, and treatment guideline from Denver. *Pediatr Pulmonol* 2022;57(2):529–537. doi:10.1002/ppul.25746

69. Sweet SC. Pediatric lung transplantation. *Respir Care* 2017;62(6):776–798. doi:10.4187/respcare.05304

70. Martinu T, Koutsokera A, Benden C, et al. International society for heart and lung transplantation consensus statement for the standardization of bronchoalveolar lavage in lung transplantation. *J Heart Lung Transplant* 2020;39(11):1171–1190. doi:10.1016/j.healun.2020.07.006

71. Wong JY, Westall GP, Snell GI. Bronchoscopic procedures and lung biopsies in pediatric lung transplant recipients. *Pediatr Pulmonol* 2015;50(12):1406–1419. doi:10.1002/ppul.23203

72. Priftis K, Anthracopoulos M, Eber E, Koumbourlis A, Wood R. *Paediatric Bronchoscopy*, Vol 38. (Bolliger C, ed.). Karger; 2010.

73. Neurohr C, Huppmann P, Samweber B, et al. Prognostic value of bronchoalveolar lavage neutrophilia in stable lung transplant recipients. *J Heart Lung Transplant* 2009;28(5):468–474. doi:10.1016/j.healun.2009.01.014

74. Radhakrishnan D, Yamashita C, Gillio-Meina C, Fraser DD. Translational research in pediatrics III: Bronchoalveolar lavage. *Pediatrics* 2014;134(1):135–154. doi:10.1542/peds.2013-1911

75. Lu B, Liu M, Wang J, et al. IL-17 production by tissue-resident MAIT cells is locally induced in children with pneumonia. *Mucosal Immunol* 2020;13(5):824–835. doi:10.1038/s41385-020-0273-y

Therapeutic uses of BAL

PART 3

13

Pulmonary alveolar proteinosis

STÉPHANE JOUNEAU, PIERRE CHAUVIN, MALLORIE KERJOUAN,
CÉDRIC MÉNARD, MATHIEU LEDERLIN, BERTRAND DE LATOUR,
ERWAN FLECHER, BENOIT PAINVIN, ETIENNE DELAVAL, AND
ADEL MAAMAR

Pulmonary alveolar proteinosis (PAP) is a peculiar, very rare disease that is diagnosed by a typical crazy paving appearance of a chest CT scan, together with a milky bronchoalveolar lavage (BAL) containing periodic acid–Schiff (PAS)-positive deposits. The classification, pathophysiology, and therapeutic management of PAP have progressed in recent years, but the gold standard treatment more than 60 years after its discovery is still whole lung lavage (WLL) (1).

PULMONARY ALVEOLAR PROTEINOSIS

Introduction

In 1958 Rosen and Castleman described PAP (2) as a disease in which gas exchange is hindered because dysfunctional alveolar macrophages cause surfactant proteins and lipids to accumulate in the pulmonary alveoli (3). This ultra-rare disease results in only 4–40 cases per million inhabitants, or 0.2 cases per million inhabitants per year (4). Autoimmune PAP (aPAP) is predominantly a male disease, with a sex ratio >2 and a mean age at diagnosis of around 50 years (5–9).

Classification of PAP

PAP cases are assigned to one of three categories (1, 3):

- Primary PAP (most frequent), caused by disruption of granulocyte–macrophage colony-stimulating factor (GM-CSF) signaling, is mainly autoimmune (>90% of all PAP), with serum anti-GM-CSF. Primary PAP also includes hereditary PAP, due to mutations in the genes encoding GM-CSF receptor subunits.
- Secondary PAP (5–10%), caused by reduced numbers and/or function of alveolar macrophages due to diseases or conditions such as hematological disorders, chronic infections, or inhalation of toxic substances.
- Congenital PAP (2%), caused by disorders of surfactant production, and so observed mainly in children.

DOI: 10.1201/9781003146834-16

PAP diagnosis

Most patients present with increased dyspnea on exertion but appear to be normal on clinical examination for interstitial lung disease (ILD). The poverty of the clinical evidence often contrasts with the profusion of radiological lesions (9).

Diagnosis is usually based on the presence of the so-called "crazy paving" pattern (septal and intralobular lines superimposed on a background of ground-glass opacity) on a chest CT scan and the presence of PAS-positive eosinophilic material in a BAL (Figure 13.1) (1). The serum contains anti-GM-CSF antibodies in 90% of cases, leading to a diagnosis of aPAP (3). A lung biopsy, either surgically or cryobiopsy, is no longer required to diagnose PAP.

Evolution of PAP

The evolution of aPAP is unpredictable and varies from spontaneous resolution to death due to respiratory failure or a lung infection. The five-year survival rate is currently around 95% (4, 7).

Secondary infections, the most common and threatening complication, occur in 5–13% of patients and account for 18–20% of deaths (3, 7, 9). Infections may be due to opportunistic pathogens such as mycobacteria, *Nocardia* spp., *Actinomyces* spp., *Aspergillus* spp., and *Cryptococcus* (1). They should be systematically screened by BAL in cases of worsening, and also during WLL with samples on both sides (9–11). These infections may even precede PAP diagnosis. Punatar et al. found that half of all infected patients showed no

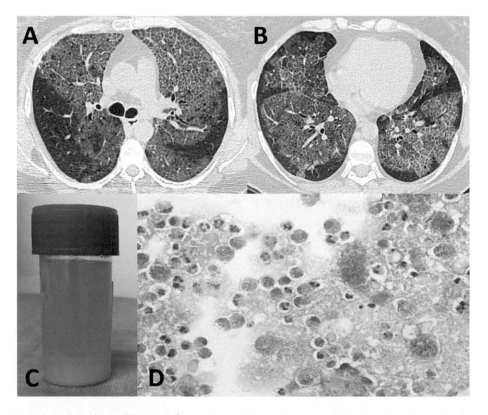

Figure 13.1 A and B: chest CT scan of a patient with autoimmune PAP showing the typical crazy paving aspect together with ground-glass opacities, septal thickening, and intralobular reticulations, sharply demarcated from normal lung. C: macroscopic milky BAL. D: microscopic aspect of BAL with large amounts of PAS-positive acellular eosinophilic lipoproteinaceous material (10).

sign of fever (11). The other symptoms of infection included a cough (64%), dyspnea (62%), and weight loss (23%). Most (75–86% of cases) of the infected sites were pulmonary, but brain abscesses were reported during nocardiosis (19% of cases). A quarter of the mycobacterial infections and half the fungal infections resulted in disseminated (lymph node, hepatic, medullary, cerebral, or ocular) infections (11).

Secondary pulmonary fibrosis can also occur, as can honeycombing during follow-up (12–14).

PAP: disease monitoring

Patients with aPAP should be followed up regularly and supervised by experienced specialist physicians. Respiratory symptoms (cough, dyspnea) and general symptoms (fever, weight loss, and fatigue) should be assessed at each appointment. Lung function parameters (especially DLCO), SpO_2/PaO_2, 6MWT, and chest radiography or CT scan (which can be low dose) should be monitored regularly, as any degradation could require a treatment change, especially WLL.

WHOLE LUNG LAVAGE IN PAP

WLL is the current standard treatment for primary PAP and some cases of secondary PAP, but not for congenital PAP (15). Ishii et al. published 51 cases of secondary PAP, including ten treated with WLL, mainly patients with myelodysplastic syndrome, and found that it was effective in only 3/10 (16).

This review focuses on aPAP, as these patients are most likely to require WLL.

Mild forms of aPAP simply require monitoring, particularly because of the possibility of spontaneous improvement (1, 3, 6, 7, 10). The therapeutic management of severe and/or disabling aPAP includes WLL, nebulization of recombinant GM-CSF, plasmapheresis, and rituximab. Lung transplantation may also be an option in selected cases.

At present, the first-line treatment of aPAP is WLL, but recent publications (15, 17) and ongoing randomized trials of inhaled GM-CSF (IMPALA-2 trial, NCT04544293) suggest that this may change.

WLL technique

Ramirez et al. first described the technique of "segmented endobronchial flooding" as a way to physically remove accumulated alveolar material in 1963 (9, 18).

Seymour et al. (9) provided a detailed outline of the method.

Following 30 mg of oral codeine, and without other sedation or anesthesia, a percutaneous transtracheal endobronchial catheter of 1.17 mm external diameter was positioned "blindly." Through this catheter, aliquots of 100 ml of warmed saline were instilled at a rate of 50–60 drops per minute. This usually initiated a bout of "45 to 70 minutes of violent coughing," which typically produced "30–40 ml of white viscid material," and was repeated four times a day for 2–3 weeks using physical positioning to direct the saline sequentially into different lung segments.

Many improvements have been made since this first description. WLL is now performed under general anesthetic. Patients are intubated with a selective double lumen intubation tube (DLT) (Figure 13.2). Left selective probes should be preferred, regardless of the side to be washed, as positioning is easier (longer main left bronchus, without the lumen of the right upper bronchus). The positioning of this intubation probe must be verified by small-diameter flexible bronchoscopy. One of the probe channels is used to ventilate the patient (protective ventilation, FiO_2 = 100%, continuous capnography ($EtCO_2$)); the other is used for lavage. The supine patient is sedated and curarized. In order to degas (de-nitrogenate) the lung, we first ventilate with 100% oxygen for 10 min., followed by airway occlusion for 10 min. until absorption atelectasis of the whole lung (19). We then instill warm (37°C) saline without N-acetylcysteine or heparin. Incremental tidal volumes of 500–1,000 ml of saline are allowed to flow into the lung under gravity. We start the outflow when inflow stops or slows significantly. The lavage liquid is evacuated by gravity ("siphoning") (6, 10). A sample of the first liter of this effluent

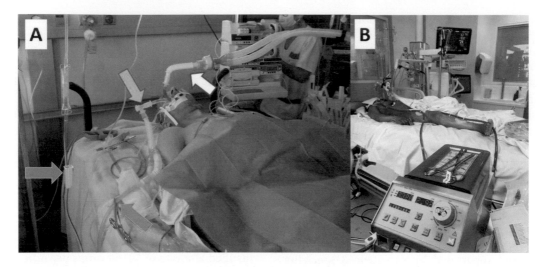

Figure 13.2 Patient admitted to intensive care unit for whole lung lavage (WLL). A: standard procedure, endotracheal intubation of each lung, one lung is ventilated (arrow), and the other lung is washed with saline (arrow). In this picture, saline is entering the right lung (arrow) and the tube used to remove the effluent is clamped (arrow). B: WLL under extracorporeal membrane oxygenation (ECMO) due to the severity of hypoxemia which could have been life-threatening with single-lung oxygenation.

should be routinely analyzed for bacteria (standard, *Nocardia, Actinomyces*, mycobacteria) and myco-parasites (*Aspergillus, Cryptococcus*). This procedure (instillation–retraction) is repeated until the effluent liquid is no longer cloudy (Figure 13.3). The more severe lung should be lavaged first (19). PaO_2 increases during the lung "filling" phase by increasing the pressure in the airways and shunting blood to the contralateral, ventilated lung (20). The pressure in the airways decreases during the "emptying" phase and blood returns to the unventilated lung, increasing the shunt and thus decreasing PaO_2 (20). Invasive hemodynamic monitoring is not required, a standard scope (heart rate, blood pressure, oxygen saturation, and $EtCO_2$) is sufficient (21). Each lung is usually

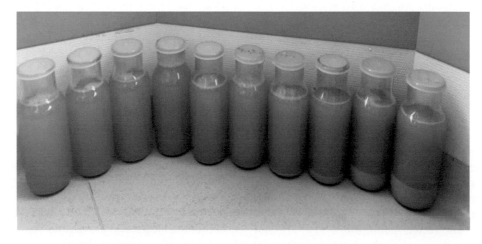

Figure 13.3 Liquid collected by whole lung lavage (WLL) (one lung) from a patient with autoimmune PAP. The turbidity and the amount of lipoproteinaceous material deposited at the bottom of the jars decrease from the right (start of the procedure) to the left (end).

washed with 12–20 L of saline, but the volume can be as great as 50 L (1, 3, 22, 23). At the end of the procedure, the residual saline is drained away and aspirated from the lung; ventilation with 100% oxygen is resumed. The DLT is then replaced with a single-lumen endotracheal tube (19). Patients are extubated a few hours later. The contralateral lung can be washed 1 to 21 days later using the same protocol (1, 3, 19, 24, 25). Patients with severe respiratory failure who are unlikely to tolerate single-lung ventilation can also be treated by WLL combined with extracorporeal membrane oxygenation (ECMO) (Figure 13.2B) (1, 19).

The WLL technique has not been standardized (3, 23) and many centers have developed adaptations to improve the quality of WLL (greater effluent turbidity) (10). Changes may include concomitant thoracic percussion (manual is more effective than mechanical), washing the contralateral lung during the same anesthesia, changing positions (alternating procubitus/decubitus) during washing, or a specific type of ventilation (repeated periods of manual balloon ventilation during WLL) (26). Segment washing under local anesthesia and flexible bronchoscopy has also been used successfully to treat patients with less severe forms of PAP. These current differences in WLL technique could be resolved by reaching an international consensus. However, all those involved agree that this procedure must be carried out by a trained team. Ideally, there should be a national reference center for WLL.

WLL indications

There is no consensus (3). The indications for WLL are set by expert centers and based on impaired quality of life usually linked to levels of dyspnea, of gas exchange (PaO_2, desaturation on the 6MWT), number of interstitial lesions on lung imaging, and pulmonary function tests (PFTs) parameters (1, 3, 19).

WLL should not be performed if the patient is suffering from active bacterial pneumonia, as it increases the risk of disseminated infection and sepsis (3).

ECMO indications are made by experts and should be discussed in the following situations: high oxygen supplementation at rest ($\geq$6 L/min?);

huge desaturation on 6MWT ($\leq$80%?), especially if this is well below the predicted values; if the patient is already in the ICU, particularly if ventilated for acute respiratory distress syndrome. It has been suggested that ECMO may be considered when the PaO_2 is less than 100 mmHg on a FiO_2 of 1 (19).

Bronchoscopy with segmental and lobar BAL procedures has also been used. However, more data are needed before segmental lavage can be considered an alternative to WLL (3).

Effectiveness of WLL

The review of Seymour found that the five-year survival rate after WLL was 94 $\pm$ 2% (9). WLL improved symptoms, exercise tolerance, chest imaging, PaO_2, and PFTs parameters (9, 22, 27). About half the patients underwent only one WLL procedure (bilateral), suggesting that the presence of anti-GM-CSF antibodies is not sufficient to maintain the disease (4). The other patients needed WLL repeated, from 1 to 22 times (9). WLL is also associated with fewer opportunistic infections (21). Smoking seems to be linked to the failure of WLL. Bonella et al. found that active smokers required an average of five WLL for remission, while non-smokers required only 2.4 (5).

It can be difficult to assess the efficacy of WLL from published data if only one or both lungs are not specified (22). We believe international experts and authors should use "WLL" when both lungs are washed, and specify "unilateral WLL," or a synonym, when only one lung is washed.

Complications of WLL

The complications of WLL are minimal when it is performed in an expert center (23). They include desaturation, bronchospasm/wheezing, pneumothorax, subcutaneous emphysema, headache, fever, cardiac pulmonary edema, hypotension, convulsion, pneumonitis, intubation dislocation (with contralateral fluid leakage), and prolonged intubation (10, 22, 27). Cardiac arrest has been reported at least once, as has one case of WLL-related death. Mortality is probably underreported (19). All the WLL-associated techniques described above (thoracic percussions, procubitus/decubitus alternations) can lead to dislocated intubation.

CONCLUSION

WLL is still the first-line treatment for clinically significant aPAP. This procedure should be performed only in reference centers with trained, experienced physicians. However, recent therapeutic advances, such as inhaled GM-CSF, may change the management of PAP, leaving WLL to be used as an adjuvant.

DISCLOSURE STATEMENT

SJ co-authored the protocol, was an investigator in the IMPALA trial (NCT02702180) and is now an investigator in the IMPALA-2 trial (NCT04544293) currently recruiting patients; both trials are promoted by Savara. All other conflicts of interest for all authors are outside the PAP field. SJ has received fees, funding, or reimbursement for national and international conferences, boards, expert or opinion groups, and research projects during the past five years from Actelion, AIRB, Astra Zeneca, Bellorophon Therapeutics, Biogen, BMS, Boehringer Ingelheim, Chiesi, Fibrogen, Galecto Biotech, Genzyme, Gilead, GSK, LVL, Mundipharma, Novartis, Olam Pharm, Pfizer, Pliant Therapeutics, Roche, Sanofi, and Savara-Serendex.

CM has received one-off advisory board or consultant fees from Bristol-Myers Squibb, AstraZeneca, and Celgene in addition to research funding from Celgene and Roche.

ML has received fees, funding, or reimbursement for national and international conferences, boards, expert or opinion groups, and research projects over the past five years from Astra Zeneca, Boehringer, Fresenius Kabi, Guerbet, Roche, and Siemens Healthcare.

REFERENCES

1. Jouneau S, Menard C, Lederlin M. Pulmonary alveolar proteinosis. *Respirology* 2020;25(8):816–26.
2. Rosen SH, Castleman B, Liebow AA. Pulmonary alveolar proteinosis. *N Engl J Med* 1958;258(23):1123–42.
3. Trapnell BC, Nakata K, Bonella F, Campo I, Griese M, Hamilton J, et al. Pulmonary alveolar proteinosis. *Nat Rev Dis Primers* 2019;5(1):16.
4. Borie R, Danel C, Debray MP, Taille C, Dombret MC, Aubier M, et al. Pulmonary alveolar proteinosis. *Eur Respir Rev* 2011;20(120):98–107.
5. Bonella F, Bauer PC, Griese M, Ohshimo S, Guzman J, Costabel U. Pulmonary alveolar proteinosis: New insights from a single-center cohort of 70 patients. *Respir Med* 2011;105(12):1908–16.
6. Briens E, Delaval P, Mairesse MP, Valeyre D, Wallaert B, Lazor R, et al. Pulmonary alveolar proteinosis. *Rev Mal Respir* 2002;19(2 Pt1):166–82.
7. Inoue Y, Trapnell BC, Tazawa R, Arai T, Takada T, Hizawa N, et al. Characteristics of a large cohort of patients with auto-immune pulmonary alveolar proteinosis in Japan. *Am J Respir Crit Care Med* 2008;177(7):752–62.
8. Prakash UB, Barham SS, Carpenter HA, Dines DE, Marsh HM. Pulmonary alveolar phospholipoproteinosis: Experience with 34 cases and a review. *Mayo Clin Proc* 1987;62(6):499–518.
9. Seymour JF, Presneill JJ. Pulmonary alveolar proteinosis: Progress in the first 44 years. *Am J Respir Crit Care Med* 2002;166(2):215–35.
10. Jouneau S, Kerjouan M, Briens E, Lenormand JP, Meunier C, Letheulle J, et al. Pulmonary alveolar proteinosis. *Rev Mal Respir* 2014;31(10):975–91.
11. Punatar AD, Kusne S, Blair JE, Seville MT, Vikram HR. Opportunistic infections in patients with pulmonary alveolar proteinosis. *J Infect* 2012;65(2):173–9.
12. Akira M, Inoue Y, Arai T, Sugimoto C, Tokura S, Nakata K, et al. Pulmonary fibrosis on high-resolution CT of patients with pulmonary alveolar proteinosis. *AJR Am J Roentgenol* 2016;207(3):544–51.
13. Luisetti M, Bruno P, Kadija Z, Suzuki T, Raffa S, Torrisi MR, et al. Relationship between diffuse pulmonary fibrosis, alveolar proteinosis, and

granulocyte-macrophage colony stimulating factor autoantibodies. *Respir Care* 2011;56(10):1608–10.

14. Marchand-Adam S, Diot B, Magro P, De Muret A, Guignabert C, Kannengiesser C, et al. Pulmonary alveolar proteinosis revealing a telomerase disease. *Am J Respir Crit Care Med* 2013;188(3):402–4.

15. Trapnell BC, Inoue Y, Bonella F, Morgan C, Jouneau S, Bendstrup E, et al. Inhaled molgramostim therapy in autoimmune pulmonary alveolar proteinosis. *N Engl J Med* 2020;383(17):1635–44.

16. Ishii H, Seymour JF, Tazawa R, Inoue Y, Uchida N, Nishida A, et al. Secondary pulmonary alveolar proteinosis complicating myelodysplastic syndrome results in worsening of prognosis: A retrospective cohort study in Japan. *BMC Pulm Med* 2014;14(1):37.

17. Tazawa R, Ueda T, Abe M, Tatsumi K, Eda R, Kondoh S, et al. Inhaled GM-CSF for pulmonary alveolar proteinosis. *N Engl J Med* 2019;381(10):923–32.

18. Ramirez J, Nyka W, Mc LJ. Pulmonary alveolar proteinosis: Diagnostic technics and observations. *N Engl J Med* 1963;268:165–71.

19. Awab A, Khan MS, Youness HA. Whole lung lavage-technical details, challenges and management of complications. *J Thorac Dis* 2017;9(6):1697–706.

20. Smith JD, Millen JE, Safar P, Robin ED. Intrathoracic pressure, pulmonary vascular pressures and gas exchange during pulmonary lavage. *Anesthesiology* 1970;33(4):401–5.

21. Shah PL, Hansell D, Lawson PR, Reid KB, Morgan C. Pulmonary alveolar proteinosis: Clinical aspects and current concepts on pathogenesis. *Thorax* 2000;55(1):67–77.

22. Gay P, Wallaert B, Nowak S, Yserbyt J, Anevlavis S, Hermant C, et al. Efficacy of whole-lung lavage in pulmonary alveolar proteinosis: A multicenter international study of GELF. *Respiration* 2017;93(3):198–206.

23. Campo I, Luisetti M, Griese M, Trapnell BC, Bonella F, Grutters JC, et al. A global survey on whole lung lavage in pulmonary alveolar proteinosis. *Chest* 2016;150(1):251–3.

24. Genereux GP. Lipids in the lungs: Radiologic-pathologic correlation. *J Can Assoc Radiol* 1970;21(1):2–15.

25. Michaud G, Reddy C, Ernst A. Whole-lung lavage for pulmonary alveolar proteinosis. *Chest* 2009;136(6):1678–81.

26. Grutters LA, Smith EC, Casteleijn CW, van Dongen EP, Ruven HJ, van der Vis JJ, et al. Increased efficacy of whole lung lavage treatment in alveolar proteinosis using a new modified lavage technique. *J Bronchol Interv Pulmonol* 2021;28(3):215–20.

27. Kaenmuang P, Navasakulpong A. Efficacy of whole lung lavage in pulmonary alveolar proteinosis: A 20-year experience at a reference center in Thailand. *J Thorac Dis* 2021;13(6):3539–48.

Index